Caring for the Caregiver

Care for yourself as much as you care for others

Linda Sage MA BA Ed(Hons)

Caring for the Caregiver

Copyright © 2017 Linda Sage (Successful Mindset Ltd.)

All rights reserved.

ISBN-13:978-1974635658
ISBN-10:1974635651

The right of the author to be identified as the author of this works has been asserted by her in accordance with the relevant copyright legislation in their country of residence and generally under section 6bis of the Berne Convention for the Protection of Literary and Artistic Works.

This book may not, by way of trade or otherwise, be lent, re-sold, hired out, reproduced or otherwise circulated without prior consent of the publisher or author.

www.lindasage.com

Disclaimer

Reasonable care has been taken to ensure that the information presented in this book is accurate. However, the reader should understand that the information provided does not constitute legal, medical or professional advice of any kind.

No Liability: this product is supplied "as is" and without warranties. All warranties, express or implied, are hereby disclaimed.

Use of this product constitutes acceptance of the "No Liability" policy.

If you do not agree with this policy, you are not permitted to use or distribute this product.

Neither the author, the publisher nor the distributor of this material shall be liable for any losses or damages whatsoever (including, without limitation, consequential loss or damage) directly or indirectly arising from the use of this product.

Caring for the Caregiver

Dedication

This book has been inspired by many wonderful caring people, from my parents, my family and my friends.

My admiration for all people who work with a caring element in their professional life and all those that show kindness to others.

My life would not be the same without them.

Learning to love yourself is the key to opening many doors.

Caring for the Caregiver

TESTIMONIAL

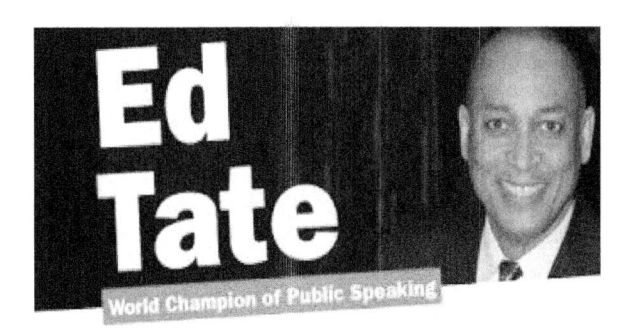

"Linda has the ability to distill an idea and make it immediately applicable.

For example, she shared the concept of "Compassion Fatigue." Within 48 hours, Based on Linda's easy to understand explanation; I was able to recognize this malady in a friend and relative!

They are both getting the help they need. Because of Linda, something I didn't realize existed; I was able to help two people in my life.

Linda has a gift for recognizing, explaining and simplifying difficult concepts.

No Fluff. No Theories. Just practical, immediately applicable answers and results."

Ed Tate
CSP – Certified Speaking Professional
World Champion of Public Speaking

Caring for the Caregiver

CONTENTS

Preface   13

Introduction   19

Chapter 1   25
How Our Mind Works Part 1
Nature, Nurture
Human Potential
Honesty
Turning Nothing into Something
Nature, Nurture, Environment
What is the Truth
Do we see with our Eyes?

Chapter 2   37
How Our Mind Works Part 2
Responsibility + Accountability = Power and Control
Valuing Yourself
Beliefs and Expectations
Beliefs and Behaviour
Why is change so hard?
What is your life like?
Are You an Expert?
Learning comes from Many Sources
Locked in to Negative People

Chapter 3   63
Self- Evaluation
Self -Worth
Self -Esteem and Change
Self -Efficacy
Forget about Worrying
Changing is a Choice at Any Age
Imagination and Reality

Chapter 4   **79**
Comfort Zones
Accepting This is How it is
Living the Life You Want
Achieving New Comfort Zones
The Here and Now

Chapter 5   **89**
Planning Your Future
Belief, Behaviour and Determination
One Word I Have Missed Out
The Vision v Current Reality
Get Ready, Get Set, Goal
The Missing Links
Last But Not Least

Chapter 6   **121**
As I Think, Say and Believe…I Am
Some Will, Some Won't, So What!
The Show Must Go On
Maximizing the Visualization Process
Good Practice Guide
Suggestions for Affirmations
Let's Get to Work

Six Years On   **133**

Chapter 7   **135**
What I have Learnt
Top 20 Must Do/Must Have
Letter to Self
Time to move on and up

Acknowledgements   **153**
About Linda Sage   **155**

Caring for the Caregiver

Caring for the Caregiver

PREFACE

Although it is true that this book can be used by anyone; I have in mind particularly caring careers and individuals who put others before themselves.

All the people who choose a professional caring role, such as doctor, nurse, health worker, teacher, police, fire, ambulance, social, work, probation, dentist, vet and many, many more; but it is not just the coal face workers, it is the Personal Assistants, the administration, the secretaries, receptionists, volunteers for charities or establishments, and carers in their own home who all put their needs, wants and dreams on hold, or a back burner for others.

The better you are at caring for others, usually the less you prioritize yourself, so it is a slippery slope of feeling unfulfilled and unhappy over a long period of time. Compassion Fatigue is another book in itself, but if you can see that you are as responsible for yourself as you are for others, your life and accountability for yourself are as important as your "duty" to others.

Taking time to invest in yourself is not to the detriment of your care receivers, in fact, it is the opposite, if you feel good in yourself, your abilities and your attitude your care giving reaches a higher level. You are less like to make mistakes, you are less agitated by smaller incidents, plus you are more empathetic and compassionate. It does not just feel like going through the motions and feeling exhausted, disillusioned and isolated. Literally, you feel like you are running on empty.

You and your goals/dreams /wishes are just as important as everyone else, it is only you that devalues yourself. Most people that choose any form of caring are already predisposed to underestimating their own worth and put their own needs and desires on a back burner. If you are willing to treat yourself this way; what message are you giving others?

Caring for yourself is not a luxury it is a necessity. However, you must believe it first, then you must action it.

If you have chosen any profession that includes a caring element, or volunteering or caring for a family member at home; you are probably already putting your wants, needs, and desires onto a back burner.

Giving of yourself to others on a daily basis takes its toll and most individuals involved in care are less likely to look after themselves. This has a negative spiral, for all involved; you as a carer feel undervalued, exhausted, and isolated. You are more likely to make mistakes, lose concentration and be easily upset or angered.

The burnout rate for health professionals is alarming, and for the most part preventable. Taking time to look after yourself, relax, refuel and redefine the beliefs that are holding you, prisoner.

Caring for yourself is not a luxury, it is a necessity; you are worthy of the best that life holds; only you do not think so. Change your beliefs and change your life.

There are lots of ways to look at life and I am not saying that mine, or what you will be reading in this book is the right or only way, but open your mind and just maybe you will find some of your own answers in my research, knowledge, views and experiences.

This book has been a long time in the making, I had been asked several times in the past, but I always found a reason to elude the question, or procrastinate enough to let the idea drop. It has been on the back burner for some time, but there are times and situations in your life that are like being hit by lightning, or what I like to call ArrrHa moments. This is one of mine.

I have talked, trained, lectured, written courses and had umpteen articles published in various countries. My audiences have been young people in schools, colleges, universities, adults in further, higher and prison education as well as the corporate and professional areas of learning and training. From one extreme social background to the other, in a variety of countries and in English and Spanish languages over a period of 30 years (where did that amount of time go!) Your mind, beliefs, emotions and actions cross all social, gender and age barriers. There are no limits to our potential except the ones that we impose on ourselves.

It has become my passion in life to share my knowledge and see people become what they had only dreamt of.

I can imagine what you are thinking now...Oh, it is ok for you, you are not in my shoes, you don't know how difficult my life is, no I don't, but neither have you been in mine and that is why I know why learning and working with this information has totally transformed my life and lifestyle.

My first statement and truth that I have learnt; is that "the truth" really isn't just that, it relies on our own beliefs, conditioning and interpretation. The truth is how we perceive it to be, not how it is. Let me just give you a quick insight here, no baby is born sexist, homophobic, racist or a bully, nor are they frightened of spiders or closed in places, but it learns in the early years things that will shape their "truth" in later life.
Potential is not measured by income, nor by the colour of your skin or the place where you are born; so I think we are

fairly safe to say that every human being is born with unlimited and unbridled potential, but whether they believe that to be true or not, has much more to do with conditioning and life experiences than their natural abilities.

If you are sceptical at this point, great, ask questions, take notes, and don't accept things as correct. There are hundreds of thousands of books, DVDs, CDs, courses seminars etc., maybe you have a few Self Help copies in your personal library. That is fine, I am not going to argue the point of them, but I hope that I will open your mind to at least the possibility; that your mind holds the key to being either your best asset, or even your worst liability.

This book is written in such a way it takes you through a variety of topics one by one, that build into each other, don't skip them or rush through them. Read each point and look at your life or areas that you are looking to change, because you are looking to change something or you would not have selected this type of book in the first place. This book will only be as good as your actions, if you skim it, or just read it then add it to the pile, then your guess is right, it will not be any different to all the others you have in the pile. But if you read it, work on the points and action them in your life, then wow there just could be a few ArrrHa moments. This is no different to going to a gym, looking at the machines, learning what they do, but you never try them out, you will not get a new shape body like that. Or, if you buy some weights and have them by your bed, you look at them every morning and night, but never start to pick them up, your muscles will not tighten that way.

There is no age limit for wanting to make changes in your life, never too young, or too old. There are no guarantees with life. We all come in the same way and we all go out when our heart stops beating. So, why are some people billionaires, and others spend their lives wishing they were.
The power of your mind.....let's see what we can unleash from these pages.

Caring for the Caregiver

Introduction

Many people will pick up a book in actual or virtual form, join interactive online training, or access an article for a multitude of reasons, but one thing is for sure that reason is important to each and every one of them, whether you want to climb Everest, be a successful entrepreneur, a great athlete, a wonderful surgeon, or the best wife/husband/parent you can be, for certain you will never achieve any of these alone. There again, nor did Edmond Hilary, Donald Trump, Mohamed Ali, Christian Barnard or my parents (who were married for 65 years, quite an achievement.)

Everyone on their way to achieving their personal or professional success have looked for and found help in a variety of forms along the way. Then, when they had reached a point where they knew a lot about their own field and had experienced problems and barriers along the way, they, in turn became mentors, coaches, teachers to the next people that wanted to achieve.

The cycle is always there, it is self-perpetuating, because people will always want to grow and succeed, knowledge needs to be shared, life, lives and lifestyle depend on it. If not we would still be living in a cave, lighting fires by rubbing two sticks together, you would not be able to read this book, nor have money to buy it, as for the comforts of electricity that we totally take for granted would still be an idea in people's imagination.

For over 30 years I have been talking, teaching, lecturing, groups as well as individuals and living my life to show people how to succeed at what they want. It is not about birth rights, intelligence, family history or abilities, not all rich people have a happy life, nor do all less financially affluent people stay where they have come from. The list of rags to riches stories is enormous, people with disabilities whether they were born with them or acquired them, going on to find fantastic success in their chosen fields. David Blunkett, Douglas Bader, Andrea Bocelli, there are more than enough names to fill a very big book. None of these people were especially talented or gifted, but they all achieve more than others with fewer impediments.

I believe that there are three main reasons behind this:

1 The beliefs you hold (particularly about yourself)
2 The type and quality of help you get throughout your life.
3 The discipline and determination you use to achieve goals

I hope that throughout this book you will see a way to work on all of these vital elements. As you progress in your own development, just as I did. You will see that outside, physical change cannot happen, until the internal programmes have been renewed or replaced.

This first step is always the biggest and the scariest, as soon as the mind is mentioned people back away, psychology, psychiatry, psychotherapy, make people put their barriers up, heads down and run for the nearest exit. Horror stories of mind bending drugs, therapies and experiments have paved the way for a lot of mistrust and disbelief that long lasting changes can be made to any areas of your life in relative ease and in a short space of time.

I have spent decades and many thousands of pounds travelling around the world going to seminars, conferences, doing courses, reading books and articles, listening to DVDs and CDs, meeting, talking to and being mentored by many of the world's experts. My journey and my learning are still going on. I am going to bring you what I believe is the best practice, know-how and insight from some of the most successful people on the planet.

In these chapters, I want to show you, that it is possible, if you put into practice each chapter, just reading alone will not do it. Read, take notes, identify areas in your life that you want to apply it to, then just go for it.......Remember it is OK to be sceptical, I even encourage it, just keep an open mind, be willing to learn, to change and want to grow, then you will get the most out of this book and you can also come back to it, time after time.

Our belief system holds the golden key to change, the beliefs about ourselves, other people, and our environment. Also, how we got these beliefs in the first place and how we can update, modify or replace them if we want to.

Our beliefs, also impact on how we look at life, what outward traits we show to others, our relationships, even our health both mentally and physically, our enjoyment of life and our habits.

High self-worth and self-esteem, (I am not talking about braggers, bullies or being bolshie) act just like a protective layer, to ward off negativity and pessimism.

Accountability, goes hand in hand with responsibility, once you know and accept exactly where "The Buck" stops and why, it is extremely liberating and powerful.

Self-fulfilling prophecies will always come true, whether **"You think you can, or you think you can't, you will be right,"** as said by Henry Ford. Human potential, there is no limit, there are only the ones we choose to put on ourselves, what we choose to learn and how much we want to develop, is truly our own choice.

The human brain is like the hard drive of any PC, the information is only as good as the programmer, if the PC is set up with a programme saying 2 plus 2 = 5, then that is the answer it will always give, until it is reprogrammed, (through advances in technology, we do see some programmes/apps thinking for themselves, but in general it is still true.) Once we have formed a habit, that is how we have been programmed, whether it is for our own good or not.

We have the capability of blocking things out; it can be anything from not seeing something around us to painful experiences, to amnesia. Everyone loses their keys at one time or another; then the more you look for them, the less you see them, it gets blocked. Then somebody comes along, picks them up and says "Are these the keys?" you know darned well that you looked there, or that they were not there a minute ago!!

As human beings we all want to be HAPPY, we are predisposed to want HAPPINESS, whether this is at the top of a mountain, the first one across a finishing line, being in love, having a child, more money, a better house, new car, taller, shorter, fatter, thinner, straight hair, curly hair, these are all illogical beliefs that outside events or people provide our happiness, which is never the case and are all doomed to failure, even if there is a short lived ecstasy, it will dwindle and evaporate. Happiness comes from within; the trick is knowing how to find it.

Progress is measurable and should be measured. I was taught very early on that a written account of feelings, emotions, thoughts, as well as behaviours and achievements, is important. Whether it is a diary, journal, or log it does not matter, but I like a Reflective Log, written at the end of each day, brings a closure to the day and helps you sleep more peacefully.

Sharing your progress with others is a great way to acknowledge to yourself what you have achieved and it can also help others on a similar path, so I always like to hear about personal and professional growth at www.lindasage.com email at info@lindasagementoring.com

Caring for the Caregiver

Caring for the Caregiver

CHAPTER 1
How Our Mind Works – Part 1

There have been so many studies, investigations and papers written on the function of the brain, they can pin point areas that function with reading, writing, physical tasks, anger, emotions and how in some people it works in different ways. We scientifically know that there are two lobes and a cortex, but just where the mind is placed is still a mystery. We cannot argue that the conscious mind is very powerful, it cannot be seen as a solid entity, but it can certainly be felt, and seen on scans as something very similar to electricity!

There is no doubt that people with psychological illnesses are not accepted, or understood in society with the same degree of tolerance as physical illnesses. We are not here to look at the depths of psychology or psychiatry, though there is no line to be drawn that individuals who are living with High Functioning Autism, ADHD, ADD, Dyslexia, Dyspraxia, OCD, Aspersers Syndrome cannot achieve results like everyone else with this book. I have worked with thousands of Young Offenders, Prisoners, SEN Pupils both children and adults. As well as with my own daughter who has four of the above conditions. There is no one size fits all with these Spectrum Disorders, each one is unique and special.

Many people who suffer with depression, any form of psychological trauma or acquired brain injury often prefer to tell people they have been in prison, rather than had a time in their life that they could not cope and needed support.

If we are all very honest not one of us has gone through our lives, no matter how old we are without some type of support, encouragement and help. This comes back to my No.2 reason, about the quality of support we receive.

That No.2 reason, also has a knock on effect with the No.3 reason, as we will learn from others the need for consistency, determination and dedication. Nowadays, many shoes have Velcro, but do you remember learning to tie your shoe lace, or a tie? Bet you did not get either the first time. In today's fast society, where your needs and demands are met almost instantly, these traits are even more valuable and necessary; after all none of us learnt anything in an instant, so imagining we can change that quickly is not logical either.

Why am I here writing this book? How come I am in a great place and time in my life and the tears, heartache, struggling and soul searching are gone? Is it luck, inspiration, ambition, talent, or connections?

Maybe it could be said to be some of all these things, but I believe we make our luck by the choices and actions we take, inspiration yes definitely from many people, ambition, of course, I want to learn and do more, talent again over these decades I have made the choices to learn and improve the skills and abilities, though when I started to write this book I had never met a publisher, an agent, never seen a book proposal layout. Connections, well I have more now than when I started all those years ago, but being in Spain for five years many of them have moved on or away. So starting from scratch again!

The difference is that I know the process works, no matter what you are looking to achieve. I have used this process to go from being a Lone Parent of a challenging two year old, in 1993 - moving back to the UK with what we stood up in - to life since 2005, living in my dream home (pool, orange trees) on the Costa Blanca in Spain.

Since the first edition of Personal Coaching for Change, that dream house split in two (literally) the insurance said it was an act of God, so no cover. I lost my mum six months to the day of moving in, within a few months I found out my partner of six years had stolen a significant amount of money from me and my parents, which lead to a very acrimonious breakup. Within a year, my ex-husband died and although in the UK we were divorced, in Spain we were still married, so I inherited 5 mortgages, and credit card debt. And, just for good measure, that all happened within 10 days of my father dying. There is much more, but let me suffice to say that, I am not saying this to brag, but to demonstrate that my continued personal and professional growth has enabled me to do this. Believe me, there were lots of up and downs along the way, even knowing all of this, they all took me a step closer to where I wanted to be and to my personal happiness. I have shared my story now with thousands of people and I have heard of many thousands more that have told their own stories of success after using this information.

It does not matter, your age, gender, nationality, or social standing, if you are not at the optimum level of personal and professional happiness, you are not the size, shape or weight you want, you don't jump out of bed each day looking forward to being you, you are not driving the car you want, or live in the house you want, or have the job you want, have the spouse you want, have the health you want, then there is room for making better choices. This process is exciting and exhilarating; there is nothing too big, or too small. It is all about you being the best you can be and feeling the best you can in your own skin. We only have one life, so better to make it a great one.

Human Potential

I want to start with my personal view on Human Potential, as far as I know with all the amazing scientific researches, scans, tests and biopsies no one as yet can measure Human Potential. I think it is quite safe to say that every single baby that enters this world has it, and as we grow it is moulded by us, our experiences, environment and lifestyle.

I think I am also safe in saying that all of us have much more potential than we are using at this very moment, no matter where we are in our lives and personal development.

I hope we can agree to start this journey into personal change that we all have huge potential. I also think it is a super power to be unleashed to get us where we want to go.

Honesty

It does not matter who you are, where you are, what you want to achieve, but being honest with yourself is often a difficulty in itself. This process is only for YOU, you cannot do it for anyone else, you cannot make somebody else change. It is personal and it has to be important to you, and important enough for you to want to change.

One of my clients wanted to lose weight, not for health reasons, not for feeling and looking better, not for more energy and vitality, not for a party or wedding, not to buy new clothes, but so that she could wear her wedding ring again.

To others that does not sound like much of a reason, but for her, it was very important, it was a big enough reason to change (and she did).

So, don't be influenced by what you think other people would be saying, find the things that are important to you. There are only two reasons to change, moving towards pleasure or moving away from pain; whichever is the stronger emotion will give you the stimulus to make the change. If the benefits do not outweigh the effort, or achievement for you; then you will not change.

Turning Nothing into Something

Imagination is like the mind, you cannot touch it, see it, smell it, but you can definitely hear it and see its outcomes. There is nothing in the world today, no piece of music, building, scientific breakthrough, medicine, play, programme, book, clothing, haircut, and the list goes on that did not start as an idea in somebody's mind.

Did the world embrace their ideas to start with.....NO, because whatever it was, meant change and change is scary. Do you remember Columbus? Nobody would back him; everyone knew that the world was flat, and he would fall off the edge! But now, in the age of air travel being more like catching a bus, we forget how he had to fight to be believed and how he could only imagine beyond the horizon, to convince not only the financial backers, but the seamen as well; as far as they were concerned they were sailing off to certain death. History has shown that his navigation and imagination, took him not to India where he thought he was bound, but to America; that is why the natives of the land got called Indians.

Imagination is unlimited, if you ask a child what they want to do when they grow up, it is all exciting things like being an astronaut, under water farmer, for them nothing is impossible, but as we grow older we reign in our imagination until it feels comfortable to us and our situation.

Imagination is not just for children, adults do dream and wish, but then we put the brakes on, so now is when you need to be honest with yourself, what is it that you really, really want, but be truthful and take off your blinkers of "Your present limitations."

Most people do not know what they really want; because they have never allowed themselves to really think about it. Your imagination creates your destination; if you can see it in your mind you can achieve it.

What do you really want: (Write it all down)

Nature, Nurture, Environment

There have been arguments, debates, articles, reports, dissertations, books, and films made on all sides of this, but you only have to look at people.

If having money and wealth was happiness, then none of the rich and famous would divorce, commit suicide, have drug or alcohol issues, which we all know is far from the truth.

If being healthy, fit and beautiful meant that life was always happy, why do models and professional athletes not have a perfect life?

If having a disability meant that you could not achieve success or independence, then how do you explain people like David Blunkett, or Stephen Hawking, to name just two of many?

If starting off from a poorer background meant you never achieved anything, then how come so many of the business moguls are where they are today? Sir Alan Sugar, Oprah Winfrey.

It is easy to stereotype people into categories, but there is usually only one person that keeps us in our category, that is our self, in the place that we think we should be.

So, we have the power to change us to be where we want to be.

What is the truth?

This is to me, one of the most interesting questions ever asked, and no matter who you ask you will get a different answer, not because people want to mislead you, lie to you or make things up, but because they actually believe what they are telling you is the TRUTH as they see it.

This is where it becomes evident that what we think is true, is actually our perception of the truth according to our beliefs, conditioning and environment. I can imagine you are now shaking your head in disagreement but, this is where an open mind is important.

One way I have of demonstrating this point is a jar of Marmite (in the Northern Hemisphere, or Vegemite in the Southern Hemisphere), yes plain and simple, same ingredients for decades, same jar, same product where ever you buy it in the world. So, the product, (or the trigger) is the same for everybody, but your personal thoughts about it vary, some are now thinking mmmm lovely on toast, others of you will be cringing at the thought of eating Marmite. So, your beliefs vary, but each one of you would stand and argue your point with a great genuine belief that the other person was wrong.

A book, or a film people read or watch, they love it, hate it, cry at it, laugh at it, are annoyed by it. The words or the screenplay are the same for everyone, but your beliefs about the content are different, so your truth about the book or the film is not always the same as others.

Sport, rugby, cricket and football is a classic of how people view, feel about and vocalise about one team or another, all due to each person's past history and conditioning. It can even vary in one household, through diverse external experience and conditioning.

When people are interviewed by police about car accidents, accounts vary from size, shape, make, model, and colour, to the number of people there were in and around the car. Not because people are unhelpful, but because they are already conditioned to the truth as they know it.

Conditioning does not need to be verbal or physical, a gesture or a huff on a continued basis is enough to etch that belief on a young memory. A baby is a blank canvas; it is like a sponge for all information, as it grows it is absorbing all sorts of information, to build the truth as it sees it, in its own environment.

Do We See with Our Eyes?

The very simple answer to this is short and sweet NO! Our eyes take in light and transmit it to the back of the eye which sends the information to the brain, the brain interprets this information and we assume we see the objects, or people in front of us.

That is why our eyes can be deceived, the magician works on this basis, they distract you and produce amazing tricks. But more than that, our brains actually see what is comfortable and right for us. How many of us search like mad for our keys, gloves, umbrellas, the more het up we get about it, the less likely we are to find them, then somebody comes along and bingo here they are.

My daughter loved the Lion King film as a little girl and I must have sat through it at least 500 times. A few years later I was at a friend's home, where her grandchild was watching the Lion King, all of a sudden the lion had the bird in his mouth, but let it go when one of the other characters told him to. I was convinced that this was a new version or a different film, as I had never seen that in the film before! It had always been there, but for some reason, I had missed it.

These are called blind spots (scotomas) and the thing is we do not even know we have them, until they are pointed out to us. We have all seen the optical illusions, some we get, some we don't; how many times have you bumped into a chair, desk, person, lamp post, door frame that you have passed a thousand times, but never saw it, until you bumped into it.

Our blind spots are not just about these physical things, but the way we perceive people to be, if you expect somebody to be rude or grumpy, you forget when they are not; anything they are nice to you about, you glide over. For example, my husband never bought me flowers, over time I accepted that;

so one day when he did come home with some flowers the first question I asked was, "What have you done?" Because what I was seeing was not coherent with the belief that I held.

How many times do we get a teenager shouting "Mum, where's my red jumper?", when you say it is on the right-hand side of the drawer, they will swear black is white that it is not, you walk into their room that has clothes everywhere in their frenzy to find this one item and you pull it out of the drawer. Then you ask "Are you blind, can you not see it" the answer is; yes they are blind and no they can't see it, just like us with the keys etc.

When we are locked into seeing something one way, we cannot at the same time see it in a different way, so you are locked into one way and you lock out anything else.

This is also a step of open-mindedness to accept that if we have one blind spot, then just maybe we have more that we just have not discovered yet.

CHAPTER 2

How Our Mind Works Part 2

In Part 1 of this we looked at the basis of beliefs, now I want to introduce you to the function of the mind, not in great depth as you are not studying to be a psychologist or psychiatrist and there are thousands of books on that in-depth knowledge (if you want it.)

I want to be able to make this easily understood as a concept, let me be clear that there are no specific areas of the brain that are named this way, but over the years it seems that people can accept and understand the concept of the way our minds work with this explanation.

Part 1 is the Conscious Mind, being awake and alert

This takes in hundreds of thousands of pieces of information and stores it in files in our brain. This is used for learning and storing; when you are in a quiz, or asked an obscure question and you answer in nano-seconds, not knowing where the answer came from, that is what I call the stored information.

It deals with information about our internal and external reality, it pulls up memories of previous experiences, so you can act accordingly, and make judgements about what is right for you. For example seeing a spider, this information goes from your eyes to your brain, the conscious mind reviews this information and compares it to past experiences, screaming, palpitations, sweating, so it activates the same system with the physical feelings, because that is how you are expected to react.

We take in information by all of our senses and it is stored, whether it is good or bad information; not filtered just stored.

Part two is the Sub-Conscious Mind, when you are resting, meditating, or sleeping

This deals with habits, attitudes, beliefs, memory, some bodily functions. Things that you do without physically thinking about them, you do not have to remember to breathe, or that you are a smoker, or you bite your nails, stick your tongue out when you are concentrating. You do it automatically, because that is you.

Part three is the Active Sub-Conscious Mind; this is the balance, which keeps you as you know you are.

It corrects for any changes in external behaviour or environment, if you walk into a room with a picture hanging off centre, you feel uncomfortable and want to put it straight. You do not have to remember that you are bad at remembering names, whenever you are in a situation your creative subconscious will make you act in that way.

It keeps a detailed profile of you, of exactly how you think you are in all areas of your life, when a situation, or somebody or something comes along and you act differently it will make adjustments for you.

If you are at a party and chatting away happily to somebody and you know yourself to be a poor conversationalist, you will do something to adjust the situation, mind goes blank, make really silly replies to questions, or spill a drink over the other person.; anything that will restore your feeling of inadequacy, so you can relax and be how you know you are.

Never underestimate the power of the creative subconscious, it is quite capable of not only making you think things, but it can physically make you sick, headaches, sweating, palpitations, feint, constrict your airway and lose your voice just to get you back to where your self-dominant image wants you to be.

This is a major combination of the "truth" as we perceive it to be about ourselves and situations. We do not act in accordance with the truth, but in accordance with our own perception and beliefs of the truth.

Here especially those people who are affected by any of the diverse brain functions as Asperger's, High Functioning Autism, ADD, ADHD, Dyslexia, Dyspraxia, OCD, they have usually been berated, bullied and diversely mentally and physically ridiculed over long periods of time. Along with an internal feeling of being different and not fitting into society generally and often into communities such as schools, clubs, work etc.

Long-term negativity throughout their academic years, of being told they are thick, stupid, disruptive, underachievers, even bad creates the feelings of inadequacy that often lead to increased levels of violence, frustration, refusal to be in certain social settings and often self-abuse/self-harm.

Even in a society of heightened awareness, isolation and rejection in an environment where academic achievement is seen as positive and good, low grades are seen as unworthy and poor achievers.

I explain the difference of the neurons in the brain that affect us all, the connections between the lobes and the cortex, if these connections like in electric wiring are strong & secure they function every time, if the wires are lose/not contacting well the light or current will be intermittent or erratic.

The deeper the beliefs are about yourself and the world, the more concentrated the task of reprogramming is. For people with limited concentration spans, this needs to be done on a little and often regime.

There is no one more or less able to choose to change; the only requirement is that you want to.

Responsibility + Accountability
=
Power & Control

This is my personal soap box, after working many years with teenagers and prisoners, the one thing that people want to do is BLAME, the school, society, the boss, the government, their parents, their peers, the teachers. This is called being a victim, a victim is weak, used, abused and overlooked. It is impossible to be positive, optimistic and a leader, when you act or feel like a victim. Being a victim you give away your power to somebody else, so if you don't care about you; why should they?

I was working in a boy's secondary school at one time and they had particular problems with pushing and crushing in corridors and on the stairs at the change of lessons. This was a huge accident waiting to happen! I asked a whole year to set an example, be only responsible for themselves walking to and from class. When others wanted to cause a scene or push into the crowd, to walk away with dignity, not be confrontational just treat themselves with respect. Be accountable for only their own actions, and how they treated others.

The first day there were jeers and name calling from other pupils, but boys in the other years started to see how these boys were walking away, they joined in. During class and registration, the participating boys sat taller, were more calm and attentive.

As the days turned into weeks, it was unusual to see any pushing or shoving in the corridors, each boy who had been involved in the fracas blaming everyone else for the pushing and shoving, now held their own power and felt much better for it.

Taking the power back, picking up the responsibility for yourself & your actions, is a big step, it is much easier in the long term than being unhappy with your life because of everyone else.

If you are waiting for somebody to make you happy, then you are going to wait a long time, if you do not care enough about yourself – why should anyone else?

The circumstances you are in now are due to the choices you have made previously. (You may deny this or believe it is not true, but really look at the choices you have made.) If you are doing things just to please others, or because you think he/she won't let me, then you are not taking responsibility for yourself. Wishing you could win the lottery, will not change your situation. Setting goals and making better choices will make the most of what you have and get you more for the future.

It was not my fault; he/she made me, Sorry I did not mean to. What a waste of your life, take the reins, own your thoughts and actions, see how different life can be. There are many social problems in society today, more laws, more prisons, tougher sentences, the problem is that the great majority of prisoners are "Sorry," only that they got caught, not that they offended, or the harm they caused to others, nor for the cost of damage. Personal responsibility is the best thing that can be taught and invested in people.

I was working in the UK Secondary Education when Citizenship was brought into the National Curriculum, to promote self-esteem and personal responsibility, what a difference personal choice can make to you and society.

We cannot always choose the events that life throws at us, but you can choose your response to them.

Response = ability that shows you can take charge and choose, rather than a reflex action that you usually do not control.

Accountability = Confidence, it is not always about being right, but when you consciously make a choice and choose to be accountable; when somebody asks why did you do that you can explain with confidence your reasons why, not a shrug and I don't know! Personal accountability builds a better world.

You can decide to make this change and to alter your self-image. If you have been looking at your beliefs that you have about yourself, how your brain acts on those beliefs, and how reprogramming that would alter your actions and outcomes.

If you are not in a place in your life that you like or want to be right now, then you need to take responsibility to change, be accountable for your future to ensure your beliefs and actions take you to where you want to be. Then you have the power within yourself to unleash the potential to attain, achieve and succeed in every area of your life that you want.

Valuing Yourself

Do you run around the house, cleaning, polishing and hoovering when you know that somebody is visiting? Get out the good china, best towels? Wear your best perfume when you go somewhere special? Keep that outfit for a wedding or party? Start the diet after the weekend, or after Christmas? Choose an educational course, but wait till the children grow up? Want to change job or career, but it's not the right time now?

If you are taking accountability for your actions, but you are not tip top in all areas of your life, maybe you are feeling defensive about valuing yourself.

I spend time with people offering them suggestions of how to address areas of their lives that they want to change, many will find as many negative replies as to why they can't.

There is never going to be a perfect, right time if you keep putting it off. When I started my qualifications in psychology and education, I had just moved back to the UK to an area I did not know anyone, from Spain (with what we stood up in), breaking up a traumatic marriage, a two year old, hyper-active daughter that did not sleep, no money, my father was ill after a cerebral haemorrhage, my mother was caring for him and going through a bad time with her own health.

I rented a small house on benefits, got two part-time evening jobs, and started my university course feeling so far out of my depth, like I was on Mars. This is where the 2nd factor comes in the quality of support; my parents could not cope with my daughter for long periods due to their illnesses. But had her overnight so I could start my course, my tutor developed my accountability for my choices. Four years later my Hons Degree Ceremony was one of the highlights of my life.

It also makes me sure that now can be the right time, whatever is going on around you, if you value yourself and your choices. Accountability for your choices goes hand in hand with self-esteem, just as responsibility goes with confidence.

The stronger your personal responsibility is for the accountability of your choices the higher your self-esteem is and the stronger your confidence is to attain your choices that you made.

What would you like to change? What would it take to change it? What do you need to do to make it happen?

Valuing Yourself gives you Responsibility, Accountability = Control & Power in action.

Beliefs and Expectations

No matter what we like to believe about ourselves and our lives, they are influenced by environment, people, places and experiences that we have along the way. Our beliefs are like our frontiers, or the outer walls of our house; these are secure lines that create our living space within that space. You can have several identically built houses in a road, the outside structure is identical, inside walls can be moved or added, but the space is the same, just divided into sections that are important to us. This is a little bit like conceptualizing the brain, the shape and size generally are the same for each person, but what it holds within it, is different for everyone.

We have previously looked at the idea of "reality" and know that it is not "truth", it is our interpretation which is moulded by our own beliefs and programming. How many of us have been bullied or name called when we were children as fat, skinny, big ears, big nose, wearing glasses, black, ugly, too tall, too short, curly hair, straight hair, poor, stupid, Muslim, Jew, disabled, disfigured in some way, slow, thick, or simply not good enough (to name but a few!)

This message hits home and accumulates even though the message is blatantly cruel or even violent, other times they are less obvious, but just as hurting and destructive.

Thankfully this programming can be deleted and replaced by us becoming "Accountable Adults", then the thoughts and beliefs from the painful experience of passing through the taunts and torment can be changed to positive helpful beliefs for us to be able to become and do all the things we really want to with the skills, abilities and talents that we have.

This can seem alien to many people, I can hear many of you saying "yeah right! It's ok for you to say," if you don't know where to start, don't worry that is where support and other people come into importance. As I said at the start of this book, nobody that has ever achieved anything, has not done it alone. I have spent over twenty-five years supporting people in finding the way to make changes in their lives, but I have also been learning along the way as well. So, my processes and knowledge have developed into a honed process of helping people change the way they think, that in turn changes how they behave.

This process has no boundaries, age, gender, colour, creed or IQ level; anyone can change their beliefs to get more out of life that they want. Not everyone wants the same things, so there is never a worry that everyone will want the same person to love, or the same job, or the same financial status, or the same body shape, the same amount of travel or the same car…so in other words, the world is not going to run out of things or opportunities because people change their beliefs for the better…..In fact, the opposite happens there are more inventions, more achievements, more financial growth globally as more people are achieving.

Beliefs and Behaviour

We have talked about how we get beliefs and we also accept that we have hundreds and thousands of beliefs, anything from I don't like tomatoes, to I love classical music, to I hate Marmite, I am a bad singer, I am a good friend the list is endless and probably you don't agree with some of mine, which is fine; because your reality and mine are different.

Many of our beliefs, we are not even aware we think them, as they are so deeply engrained "That is just how I am!" You know, the one ones like "I am not good at remembering people's names" you don't wake up every morning and think I must remember I am no good at remembering names, or I am clumsy, they are just as deeply embedded as I must remember to breathe!! They are all beliefs, which we have accepted by repeated thoughts and actions over time.

If you walked into a room today & within minutes remember everybody's name, you would feel uncomfortable because you were not acting like yourself, as you know you are. This is where the creative subconscious from the previous chapter comes into play. It will make us do something to change the situation, forget the names, call them by the wrong ones, so that we are more comfortable in ourselves.

Beliefs not only affect our behaviour, but they also affect our responses, to keep us as we know we are. If you believe you are not attractive, then somebody comes up to you and says "you look lovely", you brush the compliment off, or you think they are joking, anything other than think; yes, thanks, I have made a big effort and am pleased with how I look, because you don't believe that!

No matter how ingrained our beliefs are, they can be changed if and when we want. Maybe not overnight but the original ones were not made overnight either.

Most people have heard of a Placebo, these are also known as sugar pills. All medical trials use groups of people who have the new medication for their condition and a group of people who have the placebo, but they are all told by the Doctor that they are receiving this new medication that has great potential to alleviate if not stop their illness. Both groups of patients are monitored over a period of time, a resounding achievement for the placebo patients around 30% have a marked improvement in their health, through their belief in the "new medicine".

Most surgeons and I would say 100% of an Oncology team knows that a positive mental attitude to recovery increases successful outcomes. There are hundreds, no probably hundreds of thousand success stories about positive mental attitude overcoming all medical prognostics. (There is a list of a few at the back of the book).

It is not only the patient, but the practitioner as well who needs to remember that beliefs affect attitude, behaviour and outcome. There was a study by Success Magazine with a group of psychologists, all were asked to individually assess a group of children. They were split into two groups, asked not to confer on their assessment. One team's briefing pack about the children, told them how exceptionally well they had been doing, achieving far more than their best classmates. The other psychologists were given a briefing on the same group of children, as being disruptive, aggressive and under-achievers for their age.

It was remarkable, each group of psychologists agreed on their findings, none of the psychologists conferred with the others, individual reports agreed with the brief they were given. Their attitude had been set, they looked for traits and behaviours to support that and of course, they found them. The children were average achievers for their age, not top of their classes nor giving any educational, developmental or behavioural concerns to their parents or schools.

These are only two in a vast array of studies, evidence and stories of demonstrating "what we believe as the truth, is our own perception, which directly affects our behaviour" it is essential that you understand this, as it is a key to self-acceptance and also to any changes you want to make.

Self-fulfilling prophecies are happening every day, whether you are talking about major events, results in research, exams, or just daily life. There is nothing mystical about it; we can see it clearly by the way we think about it.

How we think produces what we perceive (all the senses), that in turn directly influences how we behave. How we behave more than anything determines the outcome we get. If we are going into a maths exam with the belief that we will not do well in this, because we believe we are "bad" at maths. Our behaviour in the exam will be stress, feeling uncomfortable, sweating; mind goes blank, even panic. The end result will probably demonstrate what we have been saying all along... A self-fulfilling prophecy.

We do it all the time, I bet the traffic will be bad, I just know I will be late for the meeting, I knew I could not stick to a diet, guess what the outcome will be........yes, all self-fulfilling prophecies; do they come true.....that is up to you.

The great thing is, that if you have positive self-fulfilling prophecies, they are just as likely to come true as well. **"If you believe you can, or if you believe you can't; you are probably right"** by Henry Ford

Why is change so hard?

No matter what we believe the "truth" to be, there is one "truth" that I think all mankind will agree on, is that change happens. Whether it is worldwide changes, such as the weather that we have been seeing in the recent years, or a change in the country you live in like the Government Leaders, or a local change such as a new office block, or housing development, maybe a more personal change, buying a new car, moving house, having a baby, getting married or divorced, a new job. The list is endless, but hopefully, you can agree on this "truth."

It is not the change that is the difficultly; it is our beliefs about the change, that cause us either pleasure or pain. As we have grown up we have been building our beliefs about our self, our environment, our life and our own worth to ourselves and to society.

If you felt loved, cherished, encouraged, surrounded by optimism; then life seemed friendly, welcoming, and trusting. Life opened up each day as a wonderful opportunity, your view of life and yourself along with your value is enhanced. If on the other hand you were left very much on your own, you learnt fear, pain and always to watch your back. Every day is a struggle to eat, survive and having you around is not helping. Your view of life and yourself along with your value is diminished.

Before we start looking at change, let's just look back a little way and add some perspective here; not so many years ago not many of us would not have been using a PC or laptop, they certainly were not around when I was being educated. My first encounter with technology was in a company I was working for, my very first job, but the central computer was the size of an office. I did not understand it and I did not stay at the company long enough to learn about it, so it was eighteen years before I was forced reluctantly into the cyber age. It is now seventeen years later and I cannot imagine my life without my laptop and PC.

There have been many changes in that time; from one side never imagining such a tool in my life, conquering my fears and frustration, to now having an amazing aid to enhance my everyday life, both personally and professionally.

As humans, we are like computers, if you think of their memory bank any information saved in there needs to be replaced to get a new response. We can reprogram ourselves and change if we want to.

Change goes on all around us, all the time, from very small elements to very big events, but it is up to each of us to CHOOSE how we deal with it. Change within our self is possible, I am not going to say easy, though sometimes it is; sometimes it is agonizing, but it is POSSIBLE. There are thousands of stories of rags to riches, hopeless to victor and victim to hero. There are millions more unwritten, the reason for the new outcome is their change of belief about themselves and their ability to change.

Most of our beliefs are no more fixed than the clothes in our wardrobe, or our hairstyle. Others are core beliefs: maybe we would die for them. Mostly we become the beliefs that we collect through childhood. As we get older and responsible for our beliefs this is where the magic of change happens.

What is your life like?

When you are looking around you in your life at the moment what do you see? This is what your beliefs say about you, your environment, your world, your personal value and the world in general that has been created. That might be a bitter sentence to swallow, maybe you need to read it more than once, maybe really being honest about your answer will take longer than reading this book.

People have shelves full of books about self-help, self-development, but unless you put into practice the new concepts, then what you are looking at around you now, is what you will be looking at around you in the future.

If you are in a constant struggle, whether it is within relationships, financially, or even with yourself (weight, gambling, alcohol, drugs), life seems to be a combat exercise, your beliefs about life are that things are hard. If you believe you can't handle wealth, or money is evil, corrupt or a mystery that you cannot solve; then you are poor. If you cannot trust or rely on people, then you feel alone.

If however, you believe that generally people and yourself are good and deserve respect, you can enjoy happy relationships. If you believe that no matter what life sends along there is something good to come out of it, then the evidence of that is all around you.

As we said previously about the subconscious mind and if your present surroundings do not coincide with the image & beliefs registered in that subconscious mind no matter if they seem too good, or too bad in comparison, a battle will go on between your subconscious and conscious mind to put that situation right. The subconscious will always win, it is determined to keep you sane, thus keeping you as you believe you are.

This is why major lottery winners, or people that come into unexpected wealth, flutter it all away because deep within themselves they do not see themselves as rich, successful people. They will feel uncomfortable in themselves and get themselves back to where they know they should be.

The reverse is true, if somebody accustomed to having a healthy bank balance and sees themselves as rich and successful goes bankrupt; they do not stay in that position long, they start a new venture and become successful again.

If you dream of, or are envious of a successful career, traveling first class, eating at great restaurants, wearing designer clothes, jewelry and driving a high-class car, but see yourself as an unsuccessful person, stuck in a job, fat, ugly, struggling to pay bills without any luxuries, do not feel worthy of being in a better place, don't really like to travel alone, or to somewhere new; how far do you think you will get?

You have the potential to be, do and to have all or any of this, the life you want. You have an amazing amount of potential, more than you know and much more than you will need. When a baby is about to be born there is not a God, Deity or Angel there saying oh we will give this one a spoon full of potential, this one a cupful and this one a bucket load, we all have it in bucket loads, but we don't realize we have.

As you look at your life right now, it is probably at the things you do not have in it at the moment, all the things that are missing, all the unhappiness around you. Then you look for someone, or something to blame for that situation, the Government, my boss, my spouse, my kids....the list goes on. STOP right there. This is where you need to be looking at your deep-rooted beliefs, are they holding you back? Were they useful once, but not anymore, many beliefs are "just because" they have always been there, or that is just the way things are. Do you have any self-imposed limitations to keep you safe from imagined dangers? Are these beliefs responsible for keeping you exactly where you are now, no matter how you try, so you will not have to deal with change?

All these beliefs are doing are sabotaging your future. They are keeping you in a place, situation, relationship that you believe you should be in. These are your limitations and self-imposed boundaries.

You Are an Expert

Change happens on the inside, from those changes inside, our outside behaviour alters, people react differently to us. This is a great aspect that changes the world; I truly believe this, and I also believe you cannot change anyone else, or for anyone else. You can help and support people who want to change and we can choose to change to adhere to somebody else. Personal choice is the key.

We all know that smoking is bad for our health, but people still do it. I know people even when they have been through life threatening illnesses and being told by an expert in that field that smoking is killing them, they still choose to smoke. Their belief is that they need cigarettes and that they are a smoker. So embedded is this belief, they see it as the truth. Whereas a non-smoker could never understand this.

Here you need to keep an open mind and be willing to question yourself truthfully; I think you will see what I mean.

We all have beliefs that compare with the smoking scenario, substitute the smoking for something else especially when the beliefs have come from judgments or opinions of others, that we have accepted over the years as the "truth.". No matter what age we are now, or our location, social or financial status, we have not grown up without some negativity to a lesser or greater degree.

How much of what we accept is up to us as individuals, we also, do not accept the same amounts in all areas of our lives. From my own life experience, as a student in school I was average (never seeing myself as a top achiever); I was good at English, Maths, Geography and History. I was very poor at art, sports and I could not sing, I was a fat child so was not Miss Popular either, just to top it all I was head and shoulders taller than all of my classmates (taking me back to average, where I knew I should be).

As I grew into teen years, I felt like the Incredible Hulk most of the time. Getting taller by the minute or so it seemed; only added to my need to make myself smaller and less significant. Though at the same time I started to work part-time as an employee I was exemplary, soon getting more and more responsibility, my beliefs about myself in my work environment became very different to my beliefs about me as a social teenager. The messages that I was receiving that "I was not good enough" were changing, this was to be the way of things for many years.

Professionally I was great at passing exams and getting promotions, confident at training and leading others, but my personal life was a mess from one bad relationship to another, the more I excelled at work, the worse my personal life and relationships got.....I did not know at the time about beliefs, blind spots, self-fulfilling prophecies, selective perception and creative subconscious. I did not even know about the power of beliefs and expectations, or how they were influencing my behaviour and of course the results that I was getting. I now understand in my own way, I was balancing out my "Average" life. Be stay as I knew I was.

When I first came across this knowledge professionally, I was very resistant and dismissive. I was sent on a course by my boss for three days, I did not sleep for a week, my head was bubbling, and so many light bulbs were going on in my head about how I had stopped myself from going forward over the years. So many situations made sense now, also knowing that there was a logical reason for the way I thought and what was more, there was a logical way of replacing the harmful beliefs with helpful ones, was like finding the pot of gold at the end of the rainbow.

It is not to say, that in the thirty years since my first introduction to this powerful knowledge that there have not been ups and downs and even some personal mountains to climb, but it has given me and still gives me a different way of dealing with events and people around me. The great thing is I am also still learning about me and the power that this knowledge brings to the lives of people.

Becoming your own expert on you, is a huge step. Taking responsibility & understanding for why you stop yourself achieving & becoming what you want, really is up to you. No

more empty dreams/wishes, just your potential to succeed.
Step 1 Be really honest with yourself about your beliefs, the empowering ones and the disempowering ones

Step 2 Be really honest with yourself about what you want, most people, in all honesty, do not really know what it is they do want.

Go on take some time here and answer these questions.

Learning Comes from many Sources

Most of us think of learning as in teacher/student mode, school, college, university. This is one form of learning; we can also learn in many other ways. Two of the ways that are often overlooked, especially by academics is the film-maker and the scriptwriter, we are accustomed to using certain books to learn from, but it is always easier to learn if it is enjoyable.

Psychology or sociology, are words that can turn even scholars' heads into panic mode, let alone somebody who has struggled throughout their school life. To me they should be the basis of every educational curriculum if we like and respect ourselves, then society would have a lot fewer problems to deal with, the prisons and probation service would not be over-stretched and without a doubt, there would be much less violence in the world.

Many film-makers are psychologists at heart (even if that is not their intent), they want to get a message out there, and they have a certain amount of time to do it, in the form of a story. Many give very powerful messages of self-empowerment out directly and also indirectly, the Wizard of Oz shows Dorothy a normal young girl wanting to live an exciting, colourful life; she thinks she needs to get away to do this, but in the end just by clicking her heels together she is in the place she started from, with a better understanding and value of herself and her surroundings. The Tin Man thought he needed a heart to be like everyone else, but his deeds and attitudes had always been to help others, so he already had a heart. The Scarecrow thought he needed a certificate to show he had a brain; he thought situations through and solved problems, long before he had the piece of paper. The Lion wanted courage, but he defended his friends, stood up to adversity and never gave up, so he too had courage even before he was given a medal. The Wizard on the other hand, pretended to have all the traits and pieces of evidence that the others wanted, but he was a fake. He hid behind glass and smoke, until finally he was seen as he really was, sad, afraid and lonely.

There are many Wizards in this world creating a lot of smoke and glass, telling people things are too hard, too difficult for them. When in fact, showing them how situations and beliefs are unfounded in a different way; a way that would make sense. People of influence as we see them, are not "Gods" they are human, they are not always right, don't ever be put off challenging a personal opinion, especially as in the cases of Dorothy and friends they already had their answers, but just did not know that they did.

It is not just fictional characters that have Negative Wizards, Walt Disney was sacked by a newspaper editor, for "not having any imagination", F.W. Woolworth was sacked for "not having any customer service abilities", Bill Gates was turned down by many banks when he wanted to finance the start of his Microsoft Company, not even every Wizard is right all the time. If these and many more like them had taken their Wizard's words as the "truth", our world would be very different today.

Listening to CDs, watching films, learning from cartoons is no less worthy, than sitting in a lecture hall in Oxford University. Unfortunately for most of us, letting psychology into our lives and learning these lessons comes at a later date in life.

Locked into Negative People

After my initial three-day course, I started to empower my life and looking at ways that I could help to empower others. I did more courses and chose to work with Young Offenders, my enthusiasm was bubbling over and with my positive Wizard head in place, and I knew I could help them make a difference in their lives. The very first group I worked with, there was a young lad of sixteen, he was living at home in an abusive environment, both parents were drug and alcohol dependent. This particular lad took to the concepts of thinking for himself and planning his life really to heart, but a few weeks into the training he came to see me with a black eye. He had tried to explain the concepts to his father, who had then punched and kicked him telling him, that there were only his rules that mattered in their house.

Whether, it is a parent, spouse, boss or somebody you see as an important person who is totally negative around you, changing yourself can be hard, but you can find the strength and the ability to move out of that environment.

This young man realized that living at home was only going to keep him in an environment and way of life that he no longer wanted, he could not change his father's attitude, nor his mother's drug dependency, but he could make a life of his own that was different. He had not finished secondary school, he had no academic qualifications but he got himself an interview with a local garage and started an apprenticeship in motor mechanics, the owner of the garage was so impressed with him and his dedication, he offered to rent him a room at his own home and help him go back to college in the evening to finish his GCSEs. By the time this lad was eighteen, he had six GCSEs and completed his apprenticeship soon after. I met up with him a few years ago; he is now a very successful local businessman, with a happy marriage and children of his own.

Was I giving these young people false hope? Was I telling them something that was out of their reach? No, not at all, Can people change? Was this a way of leaving low esteem behind? Are our negative conditioning and influences no matter how long it has been part of our lives something that we can change? Yes, 100 times yes.

No matter how destructive your environment is, or the amount of negativity throughout your life, there is a permanent way out, by using your own potential, the most amazing thing is that the more you practice this, the more success you have and the quicker it happens.

Negativity and positivity breed; just think of the people around you, in financial education they say that your income is the average of the 10 closest people to you. If you are surrounded by poor people, you will accept that lifestyle and live that way too. If you are surrounded by people with money and affluence, that is how you will live too. Positivity and negativity work in exactly the same way, but you have the choice of which one to follow!

Are all the people around you, moaning about how bad, hard, unfair life is, or are they positive and looking at ways to increase their income, improve themselves and their surroundings?

Do you like being around, smiling, happy, enthusiastic people, or are you standing around with the people whining about the boss, how your spouse does not understand you, the economic climate, how the kids are turning out? I think you can answer your own question there.

No, I am not living in la la Land or popping happy pills, but being optimistic about life, enjoying the day and the moment is so important. It is also a choice. The clock is going to tick, the seconds, minutes, hours, days, months and years are going to pass whatever we do, so why not enjoy them?
I wrote earlier about the placebo effect about belief, positive

and negative attitude about getting well, this is no different. I am not saying that all of our negative influences have come from people who have not had good intentions for us, but through their own programming and experiences, their negativity has grown into an influence for people around them.

There are lots of people that have invented things, improved our lifestyles over the centuries that were thought to be impossible things in their day, but without them we would still be writing with quills, no electricity, no telephone, no global travel, no aircraft, no running water to our houses, no railways or underground systems, no television or radio…no, I will not go on; but life today is due to the belief and insight of people who have gone before us, the inventions and lifestyle of the years to come is up to us and the generations we teach. So as Positive Wizards development and evolution will continue, and Negative Wizards will be challenged and changed.

Questions to answer:

Who have been Positive Influences in your life, what have you learnt from them?

Who have been Negative Influences in your life, what have you learnt from them?

Are you a Positive or Negative Influence for your family, friends, and community?

Look at where your own limiting beliefs have come from and how they are tied to the Negative Influences in your life.

Be honest with yourself, the answers do not matter to anyone else.

CHAPTER 3

Self-Evaluation

Self-Esteem, Self-Worth

These words have been the base of numerous studies and the roots of investigation of human behaviour for centuries. I believe that one golden key to change is our beliefs, I also believe this is the second key to unlocking personal change. Each segment is like the lock on a safe, each one drops into place and then the safe door opens, each needs to be done individually, but is instinctively interlinked with the others. If one is out of place the safe will not open,

If we identify our self-sabotaging beliefs, where they have come from, who we have been negatively influenced by; understand that we have the potential and the power to change them all to a positive and enhancing plan; then we have to know how much we are worth to our self.

Self-Worth

The value you put on yourself, in any given situation. This, of course, can vary day to day and situation by situation, but it is also related to our belief system. When you see a very famous person on a red carpet, do you think I could never look like that, or they would not look like that if they had to work like me? In both cases, you are devaluing yourself.

No, you cannot look like them because you are not them, but you can be fit, well-groomed and have good posture whatever your situation, if you think you are worth the time and investment. High self-worth and self-esteem take work and dedication, just as much work and dedication as low self-esteem and low self-worth!

Too many people have low self-esteem, for too long in their lives. If you were raised in a household where the parents had low self-esteem, then from a young age you were told you were worthless, soon you got the message into your head and you took over telling yourself, just how stupid, thick, useless you are. Unfortunately, people with low self-esteem need crutches, or support to get them through the day, so drink, drugs and violence lead to a vicious circle of repetition. People who are bullies, or demanding control in all forms of the words, is a person with low self-esteem, if they need to put people down, then they are running scared inside, they see things as a threat, so they want to demolish anyone or anything that threatens their world. They are negative people, both in thoughts and actions.

My parents were both encouraging and loving, but my father believed encouraging me meant telling me I could always do better, so I got the message "I was not good enough", this added to the fact I had been adopted, even though my parents made it a big event, that I was special and chosen, somewhere in the back of my mind I had the belief I was second best, if my own mother had given me away, I must have been bad.

Along with the "sympathy" of other kids at school, I built a belief "that I was not good enough" that was reinforced in my mind throughout my childhood with my lack of skills in sports, art and singing. You see the reinforcement does not have to be in the same belief, but others will build it up to be THE TRUTH.

It took me many years to unravel this self-sabotaging belief, but this was responsible for me keeping myself as I have said before as "average".

People with high self-esteem are the other side of the coin, they have a strong belief in their own self-worth, so do not see new concepts, or ideas, or up and coming people as threats. These are the ones that bring on new talent, as they know by the time that these people are ready to take the position they are in at the moment, they will have moved up to be in a better position too. Whether that is to do with a job, financial level, skills, education, or in a personal context.

Luckily for me, my mother was the first high esteem person who was in my life, her thoughts and mentoring were light years ahead of society and people around her. She was my first lead into set your mind to what you want and anything is achievable, again it took me many years to value her wisdom and guidance, but she knew I would get it in the end.

High self-esteem people have huge amounts of energy and enthusiasm, along with a strong sense of purpose, they are dedicated and determined. They make decisive choices as to how they want to live and what they want to achieve. They have an inner strength and calmness that helps people around them. They do not think they are perfect, or expect perfection, they can accept themselves warts and all. But know they can improve.

Self-acceptance is another key to unlocking the barriers that keep people stuck in a negative spiral. We are all human with strengths and weaknesses, knowing this you can grow out of unhelpful beliefs; then replace them with positive ones. It is not arrogance or the need for adoration, on the contrary, they don't need high-profile jobs as they are content within themselves, appreciate their lives and count their blessings every day. They like themselves and they like other people as well, for who they are and not what they have, or do.

High self-esteem is like a personal shield, you can use it to take on all the usual daily, weekly, family or life challenges in a way that makes low self-esteemed people think that they have charmed, or easy lives.

It is a personal choice, people with high self-esteem make mistakes and have errors of judgment, but they don't wallow in self-pity, recriminations, guilt or embarrassment, holding your hands up and saying "yes, I am sorry I made a mistake", "I will learn to do better". They are not defensive, moody, broody or violent in response. Low self-esteem people will take any mistake as a personal injury; they will then dwell on it, and even look for retribution.

Making the distinction between the behaviour and the actual person is an important step, because somebody makes a mistake it does not make them a bad person, high self-esteem people know this. Taking responsibility for yourself and your actions brings a huge freedom, once something is done, it is done and dealt with, you will not spend hours, days, weeks even years mulling over it and ways it could have been different.

Self-Esteem and Change

When people have high self-esteem then change is not such a threat or a risk. It is an exploration or an adventure. Low self-esteem confines you to what you know and where you feel safe, as I have said self-esteem is not like a blanket, one does not cover all aspects of our self, maybe it would be easier if it did, it is also what causes us to be individual.

John McCarthy was captured and held captive by terrorists, he endured endless physical and mental torture more than most people could ever imagine, in conditions that most of mankind would never see; his self-esteem had to be mega strong to deal with that environment and the continual threat of death. In his book, he says he was terrified at the idea of making a speech as Best Man at a friend's wedding.

A man that had lived through hell, defied death and lived to tell the tale was fazed by a room with a couple of hundred people in it. But he admits it, chooses to take on the task and has now gone on to be an incredible, motivational professional speaker.

So, never think everybody else can do things easily. We all have to work at it, to achieve new goals. Risks and mistakes all go along with this, no one became good at anything the first time they did it, you may have a natural talent, but if you do not have the belief in yourself, you will never make it happen. High self-esteem lets you focus on the wanted outcomes of the progression you are making, instead of focusing on the possible losses, or useless worrying about the "what ifs". Positivity breeds views of achievements, negativity will only focus on the obstacles in the way, and make them seem like it is too much to get over. That shield of high self-esteem will make those huge obstacles break up into small bite-size pieces.

Change is the only path forward; it in itself is the same for everyone. The only difference is the way we think and feel about it, worries, thinking of the losses, the failures and the pain of failure day after day will not be any surprise when the self-fulfilling prophecy comes about and you reinforce your subconscious picture of yourself. Exactly the same will occur when you think and feel about the positivity of the change, how it will enhance your life and all that you can gain from the progress you have made.

Change and improvement are not about potential, as we all have that; it is about the choices we are making and how we see ourselves in the new environment, if we do not think we are worthy, or we will not fit in, then we will make sure we don't. Bridget Jones films are fantastic examples of the way we believe we do not fit into places, societies or environments.

The way we know if we have high, or low self-worth is also evident in the way we talk to ourselves. Self-talk is constantly there, it is estimated that we have on average 60,000 thoughts a day. The way we know how we are talking to ourselves is the way we feel about things, positive, encouraging talk leads to happiness, enjoyment and creativity. If you are feeling sad, unhappy, unfulfilled, then your self-talk is most likely to be less than positive. So, monitoring the way we talk to ourselves is a good place to start, consciously registering our thoughts heightens our awareness of what we are doing to ourselves.

Here I would usually suggest that you take twenty-four hours away from the book and make a concentrated effort to change any negative thoughts you are having, into positive ones. At the same time you can look at the way you talk to others and how they talk to you, people that have to put others down to help them feel bigger or better, are people with low self-esteem.

High self-esteem will ease you into change, it is an effective way of losing a lot of excess personal baggage that only slows your progress down, or even ties you into situations that are not good for you. There is one additional change needed within yourself that is required for the freedom that change brings, that is your belief as to whether you deserve the benefits of change. Are you good enough to deserve the rewards that change brings, or is that all too good for you? If you believe you can't change, or you don't deserve to change then you won't, no matter how hard you try you will find a way to self-sabotage yourself. So yes, I guess in the end you will know that you have been right all along, and life will go on that way.

Self-Efficacy

Most people have heard of self-esteem somewhere along the way, even if you have not really looked into it before. Self-Efficacy maybe a new word or concept to you; it means your own estimation of your own ability to cause, make happen, bring about those things that are important to you. Also, your valuation of your confidence about your ability to learn, make good decisions and think effectively.

It also requires your personal knowledge of your ability to persist in your quest for your goals. Whether, that is learning new skills, looking for help, resources and collecting, collating information and data to get a positive outcome.

Remember how I was concerning the computer? Yes, it took me seventeen years before I created the need for the know-how and expertise, I then looked for a course and a tutor to teach me. I could have done it before, but it was not important to me then. Learning to drive, on the other hand, I passed my test within three months of starting lessons; it was a priority for me. So determination to get it done, no matter what it takes is also part of efficacy. I still do not know how to program a computer, or service one maybe I never will, but maybe it is not important enough to me to want to learn that! It is not because I am incapable of learning; I just do not choose to learn those particular skills.

Also, the great thing is, we do not all want the same skills or outcomes, so whenever we do need something or somebody new, there will always be people, courses or products out there to help us.

Strong Self-Efficacy Aids Success

Strong self-efficacy helps us to look at changes and challenges in a positive way rather than as threats to ourselves and our known way of life. Stick at the challenges we set ourselves and see them through. Find ways to tackle the challenge in the most effective and efficacious way, accept setbacks as par for the course and move on learning from that experience, to prevent similar pitfalls again. Deal effectively with the stress that change and development bring with them. Have the personal strength not to give up, or give in.

Weak Self-Efficacy will do just the opposite, hold you back and let you fold at the least resistance.

So how do we program or reprogram our own Self-Efficacy?

Mastery Experience

This grows with our own repeated success, which in turn builds our belief in our own personal efficacy

Failures, with this method, also undermines our progress

Resilience comes from a persistent effort at overcoming obstacles

Vicarious Experience

Seeing people similar to yourself succeed by continued effort raises your belief in your own capabilities to do the same

Social Persuasion

Raises your belief that you have what it takes to succeed, your activities are structured in a way to success

Physical and Emotional States

Efficacy is increased by improving your physical state, reducing stress, or learning how to listen to your body and mind. A positive mood strengthens your perceived efficacy just as a despondent mood decreases it.

So, I hope you can see how these three particular sections are linked together, but work on each section is required.

Self-Talk, triggers your feelings and emotions, which in turn causes your behaviour to fit with your beliefs. Self-esteem is your value of your worth to yourself and others, which affects the way you talk to yourself, self-efficacy will mirror your self-esteem (your value) reinforcing your beliefs about your own abilities.

When you go through events and experiences in your life, you do not just remember the event or experience, you also record the emotions and behaviours that went with them. That is why all of these are so intertwined but also individual.

Mastering your Self-Talk is the third key. So, for the next 24 hours; no put-downs or negative views about yourself, consciously change those thoughts and see how much better you feel about yourself and how you can strengthen all of your beliefs about yourself, in turn, your positivity will breed positivity in your outlook and behaviour. See how many people notice the differences in you.

Forget About Worrying

What happens when you worry, is it anything positive?

Ok, we all worry at times, but there are people out there who spend their lives worrying about things that have not happened yet, and about things that have already happened, both of which we all know logically we have no control over at all.

Many people have looked into and investigated all ways to look into the future, so far to date, no scientific data can support any of the findings, time travel has been the theme of numerous books, films and theatre plays. Worrying about a future event is a waste of our time and effort. Likewise, we cannot change a single thing about the past, but we can accept it and learn from it. Worrying about the past, or the future is only reinforcing doubts, fears, injustices, and generally negatively affecting us mentally and physically, sleep deprivation being one of the negative side effects of worry.

People even worry about events or activities that may never happen, but just in case. Prolonged or constant negative strain on your body and mind can lead to stress, depression, fears, phobias, illnesses (how many ulcers and heart attacks have worry as a key component) we have already looked at how our thoughts cause our behaviour, so extensive negativity within our system is going to cause meltdown in the long run. Mind and body are combined, they generate effects and conditions.

Worry in itself is negative; it conveys an instant idea that something has to be wrong. Many people try to imagine the worst a situation can be, then anything less than that is a bonus, but if they are already looking for the negative outcome, then that is what they will find. We also associate worry with a way to show we care, telling kids to be careful, take care. We send them out with negative conditioning already planted as a belief. The next generation is already being programmed.

I spoke earlier about the positive effect on illness and recuperation with a positive attitude, stress, worry and pessimistic thoughts are not going to get you to where you want to be, but they can keep you where you don't want to be.

Changing is a Choice at any Age

As children we are undoubtedly influenced by our environment, parents, teachers, peers, television, etc. etc. but as we grow up we can take charge of our beliefs and lives. Becoming accountable for yourself and our own life, is a choice everybody can make, but it is a personal choice, for some of us it comes earlier in life, for many we have to go through an array of traumas, events, heartache and pain before we learn that there is another way to do things.

Each time you have positive thoughts, or change a negative thought to a positive one, the positive action enhances your personal power, making the scales tip to the positive side. I am not saying that there will be no difficulties or sadness in your life. If you focus on the positive outcome, the solution rather than the problem, you will have more strength to deal with whatever life deals you. By concentrating on the solution and outcome, you are not overwhelmed by the problem.

Look at what you want, rather than keep thinking about what you don't want. Remember back to the first steps.

Step 1 Be really honest with yourself about your beliefs, the empowering ones and the disempowering ones

Step 2 Be really honest with yourself about what you want, most people, in all honesty, do not really know what it is they do want.

Then move towards the life, love, lifestyle, income, body, health, fitness or whatever it is that you want.

Imagination and Reality

As children we are encouraged to have imagination in games, most of us have had imaginary friends, but as we get older our imagination seems to get reigned in and we have to conform to expected standards. I am not saying that living to expectations is a bad thing, but it is when you are conforming to expectations of others, or the created expectations of what life is about that is not making you happy; then it is a bad thing.

Our mind and imagination are not bad things. They are effective and powerful, but they can be confused and mislead, for good or bad. How many of us have been on fairground rides, that are inside a capsule, but as the film rolls and the seats move we are convinced that we are in a dare-devil racing car, helicopter, or skiing down a mountain side at mega speeds, you feel the adrenaline, your pulse races, the pit of your stomach drops as you see the ground disappear from under you; you grip on tight to the safety rail, or the person next to you. Though logically you know you are not in danger or in those places, but your sub conscious mind does not accept that, it believes what it is seeing and your body reacts to that stimulus.

The same is done in athletes, pilots, and astronauts training, they cannot keep crashing planes to practice for an emergency; athletes run the race in their mind, so that their bodies are ready when race day comes. We do not need to actually be in the situation we want to be in, we can imagine it, and then when the sub conscious picture is stronger than the reality picture we are empowered to achieve what we want.

The stronger we make the picture, the more details, colours and smells, the more real it will be. Cut out pictures from magazines, in these days of computers you can make your own movie of how you want your life to be. We have been programmed by people throughout our lives, we have accepted their "expert" view as true, so now taking and accepting responsibility for our own beliefs, means reprogramming. It is not immediate, but it is effective, I cannot give you a magic wand but these effective tools can improve and enhance your ability to accomplish all your goals.

Don't be hard on yourself and building your self-efficacy will build on hic-ups and detours, it is an ongoing achievement. We do not wash once and expect to be clean for the rest of our lives, we expect to wash on a daily basis, more sometimes when it is hot or we go out somewhere special. This process is the same, building a new reality of how things are; you need to be embedding the pictures at least on a daily basis, more than once a day is also great.

Listen to the positive voice you are cultivating, yes I can do this, yes it is possible for me, yes, I will make the change. When the negative thoughts pop up, don't ignore them, or get angry with them, just say ok that was how I was, this is how I am now, just change them to the positive. Believe you are worth the effort and you deserve the great things that you want.

Today is never too late to start. Whoever you are and whatever you want, the first step is to know it, want to change to be able to get it, see yourself in your new life and believe you are worth it.

Caring for the Caregiver

CHAPTER 4
Comfort Zones

From babyhood we are introduced to "Comfort Zones," for a baby it could be a dummy or a thumb, to get them relaxed and to sleep. As the tot gets older it has a blanket, or a favorite toy that it clings to, the world of a baby has confined spaces, a cot, pram or arms, the world opens up as they start to crawl and then walk. Once they are at school, they start with hobbies and comfort areas of their own, these develop as they grow.

Our areas of comfort widen and change throughout all of our lives, we can purposely choose to change our comfort zones, to do things that we are not accustomed to, in places that we are not regularly in, by just dropping ourselves into it – sink or swim attitude, or we can push the boundaries as we grow. As human beings, we need to grow and the only way to do that, is by change.

Have you ever walked into the wrong public toilet in a bar or hotel? When you realize you soon feel very uncomfortable, you physically react by wanting to get out as soon as possible, you feel embarrassed, go red and even sweaty, you are in a place, you do not belong. You know it and feel it. If you have ever been to a football match and got into the wrong area, the feeling is very intense and takes away much of the pleasure of the match. It does not have to be as intense as that, just put your coat on with the other arm first, or put your shoes on the other foot first, or try crossing your arms the other way round, it feels wrong for you.

When you want change in your life then your comfort zones have to adapt as well. Our reactions to where we feel comfortable can enhance our lives or they can be limiting. All phobias are limiting beliefs and minute comfort zones, once your home could be your castle, but it could also be your jail if you are agoraphobic, your mind limits your physical boundaries. It is not all in your mind, because you feel physically sick, stomach knots and your legs cannot carry you; it does not have to be like that.

Our comfort zones go hand in hand with our beliefs about our self-esteem and self-efficacy, these are all like pieces of a jigsaw that make us up as humans, they make us individual and they are not permanent. Generally, people with high self-value have wider comfort zones, and as a rule of thumb people with low self-worth tend to have narrow comfort zones. When you value yourself and you accept that sometimes you fail, then nothing is that limiting. Fear of failure and fear of rejection, are two major limitations for us and our actions, for many people it is better not to try, than to deal with the failure.

Making ourselves feel comfortable is a fundamental human need, once again we can have very wide comfort zones in one part of our life and very narrow ones in another area, so when we are looking at personal growth it is a good idea to get a rounded development, by that I mean there are some people that devote all their energies and development to their career and their personal life is in tatters; there are others who have great relationships, but are ill and broke all the time, this is not a balanced life. They have wide comfort zones in one area and very small ones in other areas.

I spoke about the imagination and reality in the previous chapter and we can use the same techniques with your comfort zones, imagine yourself in that situation, find ways to experiment, when you learnt to swim did you just jump in, or did you first use floats or a rubber ring? Learning to ride a bike, did you start with a trike and then move on to a two-wheeler with stabilisers? Every situation can use the same techniques, when you are teaching a child to swim do you talk to them of the dangers of the water, or the benefits of being able to swim? The same goes with a bike do you take a child to a main road to practice with lorries and cars flying by them, or do you use a quiet garden or a park?

There is nothing new here, we use these methods and techniques in life, but when we are adults we tend to forget and expect ourselves to be able to adapt without preparation.

If we were all able to accept change without any fear of failure, how much more would we be doing?

Caring for the Caregiver

Accepting This is How it is

It does not matter if it is a New Year, new car, new school, college, university, new job or new house, it could be a new partner, spouse or business. When something is new we see it with a wider vision, but as we get used to it, more comfortable with it, as we know it. For example, when you first buy a car, you wash it and clean it regularly, no eating, drinking or smoking, but as you get used to it; snacks and dirt start to enter, the car gets washed less and less, you don't seem to see or mind the mess, the smeared windows or the mud splashes along the paintwork. You don't even see it, you build up a blind spot to it, you feel comfortable; until your parents or your boss want you to pick them at the airport and all of a sudden the car screams at you, yuck, what a mess and off you go cleaning inside and out. The mess was good enough for you, but not good enough for others. When you want to sell the car you clean it and keep it clean for people to see, so the best value of the car is seen by all.

When we become accustomed to something that builds a comfort zone, whatever you are accustomed to earning, you get accustomed to spending and when something comes along to change that, either by losing your job or getting a promotion, it will require change and adjustment, how will you fit into the new zone? You will need to either, take up the challenge and replace the income that you have lost and are use to, or you accept less and live that way. With the promotion you can invest in a new wardrobe to fit with the position you now have, you can learn more skills to keep adding to your career prospects, you can become accustom to a new status, or you can feel so out of place, so inferior that you will be clumsy, accidental and makes errors in your work, then soon you will be back where you feel comfortable.

This feeling is easy to stimulate when you are out and about, if you are not accustomed to frequenting the Savoy or Ritz hotels, when you have an opportunity to visit either, you will feel as if everyone is looking at you, and feel physically out of sorts and out of place. So, next time you are in one of these places and you want to feel comfortable in them, walk in and take in the environment, see how people are that feel at ease there, so you can see where you need to change, to be where you want to be.

Living the Life You Want

Life is amazing, or it should be. If you are not living the way you really want to, if you are not happy with each day, then there needs to be a change, you can wait and make excuses as to why now is not a good time, but there is not a single time in your life which is the perfect day for change. It is however, the perfect day when you decide it is the day, no matter what is going on around you.

There is no change without risk, there are no guarantees, but by changing your attitude regarding change makes it a lot easier. It is probably no surprise to you to know, that to rise above others is risky, just like each and every person that has gone through change has found out. Are you worth being out of the ordinary? Do you see where the self-talk, self-esteem, self-efficacy, comfort zones all come into play here the higher and stronger they are, the easier changes seem to be, the lower they are the more you struggle to get out of the rut you find yourself in.

Just before you go running off to the horizon, let's just look at an average life, we have all grown and changed in our lives already, we learnt to walk, leaving the safety of our playpens or cots. We all went to school so leaving the comfort of our home and being all day without the constant comfort of your mum, learnt to roller skate or ride a scooter and a bike, you have been for a variety of interviews and secured a college/university/job, you have met "somebody special" at some time and been brave enough to hook up with them (even if the relationship did not last) all of this by our own effort and acceptance of change. So you already know how to change successfully, and that you have the potential to do it.

On the other hand, some of the changes that we have taken on before may not have been so successful, whether that has been in a romantic relationship or several, each time you have chosen to try a life with a person which has ended in sadness and hurt, maybe a marriage in divorce, or being made redundant, the memory of the turmoil, hurt and pain start to outweigh the happiness of achievements you have felt on the successes you have had. So, we build up a balance of bad experiences and this makes us less likely to embrace change, by focusing on your previous successes you will build up your own confidence in your ability to achieve successful changes in your life.

Achieving New Comfort Zones

As I have said previously, there are two ways to widen your existing comfort zones. Jump in with both feet; we can do this at times; it is not a great recipe for success as the stress and strain that this method causes over long periods of time can be detrimental to your overall health and wellbeing.

Visualisation, is well documented as a way to see yourself in your mind whether in the subconscious or conscious state. Just think about the surround sound and surround vision movies, the digital and high definition age brings to life the story and makes us feel as if we are part of it. Taking the time to reprogram your own picture to what you really want, how you want to live, make it your own vivid reality and you will work towards making sure you live that way.

The Here and Now

Now is a good place to start, one term I like for this is our "Current Reality", this is who we are and where we are at the present time. In consistency with self-fulfilling prophecies we are now what we have been thinking of and acting like in the last few months, if we change today the way we are thinking and acting about something in a couple of months' time we will be doing something different to today.

Reading this book is a step; if you were not interested in change, you would not be interested in this. Are you still like a butterfly flitting from one book, website, DVD, article, webinar to another, or are you ready to sit down and actually start to do something about your new future?

There are more Chapters to this book, but before you carry on reading I would ask you to stop here and actually do what has been written about up to now. Make your blurred dreams/goals into a format for a future reality.

Start with your current reality, what are you happy with and what do you want to change?

Make two lists, perhaps write them in a note book, or open a file on the computer. Then go back and number them from 1 to whatever in the importance to you. The items you do like in your life are as important and the areas you don't.

Once you know what you want to work on, then think about what your self-talk is like in those areas, make sure you change the negative to positive. Look at the positive ones as well and see how good you are in those areas, this reinforces your belief in your own ability to be able to succeed.

Then look at your beliefs, which ones are keeping you in the places you don't want to be?

Write them down and then rewrite them in a positive form that will help you move towards the outcomes that you want.

One word of warning: don't blame, or beat yourself up about any of the points, here you just want to identify and change them. If it is your first time doing this, and you are having problems finding anything you like about yourself or your life, you can ask a friend (that you trust) what they think. Remember, it is only their opinion of you, but it might help you start to look at yourself in a more objective way.

What would your perfect day, home, partner, business, car, holiday, job, be like? Don't be tempted to cut corners and accept second or third best. What do you enjoy doing? Why do you get up in the morning? What would you try, if you knew you could not fail?

If your get upset, or even angry when you are looking at your life, that is fine as you are opening up dark places that up to now, have been holding you back. We build up the blind spots to make us feel comfortable, we minimize our comfort zones to stop ugly memories coming in. But remember that shields to keep hurt out, also keep us in.

Then look at how you value yourself (self-esteem and self-efficacy) in each of the situations you have identified that you want to change. By now you will be seeing a pattern emerging. Maybe your areas of change are linked; try to ensure you have a balance between all areas of your life.

This will take time and effort, don't try and do this when you are tired, under the influence of alcohol/drugs, or emotional; also it doesn't need hours and hours at a time as it can be emotionally draining. Remember about keeping clean, you wash every day, this is a similar process. I would suggest that you put on some happy music, dance about and get your excitement and energy level high, you will be able to look inside yourself with greater clarity. Also remember, there are no right or wrong questions to ask yourself and no right or wrong answers, just be honest with yourself,

Maybe you are thinking what's the point; I'll just skip this part. That, of course, is your choice, as is all change and development, but if you don't know what you want to change and what you want to change it to, then in a few months or years to come things will be just the same as they are now. This is like buying one of those keep fit DVDs/Apps, you buy it with all good intentions, you play it through and may even do a bit on the first time, but then it gets unopened. You have the tools and the potential, but not the determination and self-faith, then you will say yes, I have that DVD/app or that book and they have made no difference to me. Participate and they will give you an outcome.

Once you know where you really want to be in specific areas of your life. Read on and see how we can get you there. The future you want, is closer than you have ever thought.

CHAPTER 5

Planning Your Future

Your Own Action Plan

This is the process to pull all of your hard work together into a solid plan. One of my first mentors always hammered home to me; a very old, but worthy phrase. *Failing to plan is planning to fail.* It is as true today as it was then.

Why do I need them? Goal Setting is literally like drawing up your personal blueprint for your life, your future.

Human Beings are teleological, meaning that they can function in three ways, just like an airplane;
1. Controls, guidance and destination
2. Autopilot
3. Drifting.

1. Controls, guidance and destination.

A pilot, planning a flight, would lay out a map of the world and plot his route from departure to destination (even in these days of computers and GPS). If the distance was too long he would break it up into segments, to refuel, or take on supplies, or even to have a rest. In the planning stage, things like time, speed, distance, etc., are considered to reach the destination in the best possible condition.

During the flight the pilot uses the rudders to compensate for any deviations to his route, to increase or decrease his speed if he hits turbulence or a tailwind. To give his passengers a smoother, more pleasant journey.

2. Autopilot

The pilot can use autopilot on some stretches of the journey, to have a short break, to help concentration, but is watchful of the monitors at all times.

3. Drifting

Drifting occurs when the wind changes direction or even strength, the pilot is aware of this vigilance is required at all times to read the equipment all around the cockpit. Adjusting the rudders to keep on track, just one degree deviation gets wider as the aircraft goes off in another direction, and could end up on a completely different flight plan, the destination could then be on another continent. Imagine how unhappy the passengers would be then!

Controls, Guidance and Destination

As we set out on a journey through life we can choose our destinations, some might just be like one stop on a bus, and others will be like a short flight and some even halfway around the world. Setting out our goals for what we want to have and achieve, can be in long term and short-term goals, the short term goals are like stepping stones across a river, or the stop-overs on a long haul flight. To achieve the goals we may need to take on more responsibility, or new information, we may need more or new skills, all of these we can see when we plan our journey.

Autopilot

This we also have, where we let the subconscious mind take over, we go through the motions, but are not really there. So we cannot see anything along the way and we cannot see obstacles coming up. Also, by setting out our goals, and then just putting them on a shelf, thinking that we will remember all about them in the time to come.

Drifting

Some drifting is expected as we are learning along the way, but just like the pilot if we are vigilant we see the change and compensate back into the direction we were headed.

The worst case of drifting is when goals are not definite the first obstacle or person comes along and sends us in a different direction, we let our goals go, to fit into somebody else's goals. Then, just like the aircraft, we can end up in a totally different destination to where we wanted to be.

Making the effort and having the dedication to decide what it is you really want, then write it down, take the time to visualise about what life is like having achieved your goal, not just once, but on a daily basis, even several times a day to reinforce the new image in your mind. To put yourself out to learn new behaviours and skills to enhance your new achievement is not for everybody.

Educational studies show that 97% of adults do not plan their life, they plan a journey, holiday, party or wedding, but all areas of their life they leave to chance or fate. So, is it so surprising that the same studies show that overall the 3% of people that do plan and know what they want out of life actually own 97% of the overall wealth of the study group.

My first mentor Richard Dunhill embossed in my brain the need to plan and every mentor I have working with since has done the same and I have no doubt all the ones in the future will do so too, just as I have done with hundreds and thousands of students over the years.

Write out your goals in details, not just I want a house. What type of house, where is this house, what colour is it, type of windows and doors, what is the garden like, how big is the kitchen and the bathroom, how many bedrooms, what colour carpet, know every detail.

A year or so after moving to Spain, into my dream home, that I knew needed some renovation work; which I had planned and drawn out myself, the house suddenly split, the whole of one side of the house subsided. My dream was shattered, but I revamped my goal and my drawing to rebuild the house. I had never done it before, never even imagined it, but in eight months I had my new home. During those eight months anyone I brought to see the demolition site I would walk through the house saying this is going to be the kitchen and describe it in detail right down to the tiles and new stainless steel kettle and I did that with every single room and the garage for three cars. My goal had to change because of an obstacle, but I kept my eye on what happened, and then compensated. To create the outcome I wanted.

When you do plan your life and work towards your goals on a daily basis, you can chart your successes, watch your progress and confidence in your own abilities grows. A newly qualified pilot would not be setting off on a long haul flight on a jumbo jet to one of the most difficult runways in the world, so don't be hard on yourself if you want to test the water. Write out some long-term goals and break them down into short-term ones to measure your progress.

Tell people about your goals as you are reinforcing them to yourself as well, they might also know somebody that could help or support you in some way. If people laugh at your goals, don't get upset or embarrassed, just think how good you will feel when you achieve it and prove them wrong.

Belief, Behaviour and Determination

Yes, you have seen this heading before when we were looking at our beliefs and how they help or hinder us, how that has a knock on effect to how we behave, but here it is the same principle applied to our goals, believe in your goals, behave as if they are already achieved and be determined to see them through.

We are extremely high functioning individuals once we set our minds to something, we can collect, store and use information about whatever we want to get the outcome we choose. Our own mini satellite dish in our brain is super-efficient at collecting information and filtering out the rubbish. This system of cells and neurons are called our Reticular Activating System (RAS) which is our safeguard mechanism as we could not possibly deal with the amount of information all of our senses are taking in throughout each and every day, it would simply overwhelm us. That is not to say that threats to you will be removed, the RAS is also a protector.

So locking onto information that is relevant, useful, enhancing and also inspiring and locking out information that is destructive, unhelpful, depressing and disturbing enables us to achieve goals and outcomes. When we set a goal it is because it is important, relevant and desired by us in our life. This raises its importance and makes you more aware of it around you. Have you ever noticed once you have decided to buy a certain car after much deliberation, your mind is made up: then all you see are those cars everywhere, giving you the good information that many people just like you, have made a good choice in buying that car.

Once you have set your goal to buy a car, you then find out about the cars, even test drive them, you decided and make your choice, the determination then digs in to get you what you want. Nothing is achieved without determination, you can have skills and abilities naturally depending on the goals you are setting, but even the best amateur sports person does not make it as a professional without learning more and practicing more. If you are determined to achieve a goal it means you will do whatever it takes, you will go the extra mile to ensure you can be triumphant.

One Word I Have Omitted Until Now - HOW

No, this is not an oversight, I am guessing you have raised this word many times in your own minds. How am I going to change my choices, beliefs, self-talk, self-esteem, and efficacy? How am I going to reach a goal that is miles beyond my current reality?

This was done on purpose, because we limit ourselves with a HOW Goal. ... I really want to fly to Canada Business or 1st Class, sounds great, but I am broke; so how am I ever going to do that!! Thinking like that you probably won't achieve it, as it is a dream or a hope, you do not see yourself as worthy.

I don't know how nor do you, but when we set those goals, have the belief we are worth it, and visualise it, we make it happen. I am not going to get all mystical or philosophical here, but there are laws, gravity is one of them, nobody will argue that what goes up will come down sooner or later. There is also the law of attraction. Whether you believe in the universe or a God or a Deity it does not matter, what matters are the thoughts and energy that you are emitting, because that is what you will be drawing back to yourself.

Remember RAS, if you are actively looking for something, you will find it; you will draw to you the information you need. We know by proven scientific research that we have our own electrical force, all the medical scans use that to tell us how we are health-wise. If you have been by a car or connected to a live electricity cable you have felt the connection, or rubbed a balloon on your hair and then placed it on a wall or ceiling, we put enough charge into it to keep it in place.

How; is limiting and puts blinkers on us, we are resilient, resourceful, powerful people, never underestimate your own ability to make your own world just exactly the way you think and believe it should be.

See the end result of your goals in as much detail as possible; add determination and a positive attitude then you have nothing to hold you back.

When you are new to this be careful there are many people out there that want to burst your bubble, and they will ask "How are you going to do that?" "Where are you going to get the skill/knowledge/finance to do that?" "Where have you got ideas like that from?" You will feel under pressure and falter saying and thinking "I'm not sure, I don't know" then you go away and think "It can't be done, I must be mad". WRONG, no matter what it is that is important to you, it can be done. There have been people that have gone before you: look at their stories, there is always a different way to do things; than the way you have always done them.

No one has started any new venture without somebody trying to burst their bubble, but their vision and their belief and determination found the HOW. The only important word here is WHY, when your reason to set the goal, or the outcome you want from that goal is paramount to you, you will find a way to do it. Enthusiasm, passion and determination will blow any 'HOW' out of the water, when you are an end result person.

I have had many people tell me what they think I can and I can't do, in some past situations I have been swayed by opinion, but really it was my own choice and lack of belief, dedication and resistance to see through my own goal. We don't have to be talking big goals here, it could be something simple like I started my healthy eating and exercise plan, visualised my new shape and am doing well, starting to feel the benefits. Then a friend pops in for a chat with a bottle of wine. Do I open the wine and share it with her, thank her and put it in the fridge, offer her only water because that's all I am drinking, or offer her a glass of wine and be happy with my glass of water?

Many times people will say, "Go on its only one glass" but this is where your value of yourself, your determination to achieve your goals comes to the test, what is more important to you. The outcome with your shape, or pleasing a friend? Whichever you value more will win.

The power, potential and abilities you already have, all you need to do is channel them to what it is you really want, visualise it and know you deserve it; then nothing will deter you from achieving it; because you will find a way to be triumphant.

The Vision v The Current Reality

Previously we have identified what your current reality is, where you are and what you are today. The vision you are creating with your goals is what you are planting and nurturing into your subconscious on a daily basis, at least once a day (more is better), so that you can see, feel, smell, hear and touch the reality of the new life that you want.

You may be thinking that is ok, I have looked at the way I talk to myself, I have looked at my sabotaging beliefs and at my self-fulfilling prophesies, but nothing is changing. This is where you need that added ingredient of energy and drive. We are so capable and amazing that we make it all happen naturally.

Have you ever been in a room where a picture on the wall was not straight, did you feel the need to straighten it? The longer you looked at it did the feeling get stronger? Did it even stop you concentrating on other things because it was "out of place"? Did you have to resist the urge to get up and straighten it, or did you give in and make it right? This is called Cognitive Dissonance, Cognitive is anything to do with thoughts and Dissonance is out of order or out of sync.

The most famous name for investigation into this field is the Gestalt Therapy, there have been enormous researches into the thought process of when our surroundings are not as we imagined them to be, the mind is amazingly apt at moving the body to compensate and make it right.

Do you remember the idea of Comfort Zones and going into the wrong public toilet, or the wrong end of the football match, our mind realizes that we are not in the right place for us, and then causes us physical symptoms to change. This is where we gain the energy, and enthusiasm to make our external picture the same as our internal one. We get the drive and ambition to change.

One word of caution here, a common error with goal setting that people set their goal, get all fired up and reach them, them zap – lethargy and let down, only because goals are not a one-time investment, as you are progressing towards your goal, you want to be setting the ones beyond that and so on. That way you will be fired up and ready to keep climbing and achieving more and more.

Many people plan their wedding, in every minute detail, they even book and think about the Honeymoon, usually not in as much detail, but how much detail do they give to after the Honeymoon to living their daily life as a married couple? So, after all their goals or dreams have been achieved on their wedding day, how many arguments happen on the Honeymoon? When the happy couple comes back home to everyday life, it feels like a come-down. But, if they sit and build goals for their life together and their individual goals, the enthusiasm and the energy return because they are on a new path to achieving.

The old saying goes "always ask a busy person to do a task", the more you do the more you can do, self-fulfilling prophecy or reality. Have you met these people that are like buzzing bees, here, there and everywhere. They have passion, drive, enthusiasm and energy when you have goals and deadlines; something that gives a time constraint on all you need to achieve....you can do it. When you decide oh it can be done anytime, that is a job that never gets done, or a goal that never gets achieved.

Sad to say it works the same the other way, a lack of goals leaves you exhausted, tired, emotional even bring on depression. Lying about on the sofa with nothing to do, when you get up you ache, your joints creak and your head is often heavy. Our bodies are made to be vertical, not horizontal, we heal and live better on our two feet. Yes, we need rest, but lounging about without any direction is not rest. When we have been busy and achieving things throughout the day how much better do we sleep, how much more do we enjoy putting our feet up just for a while, that is relaxing.

Also, it is how we see ourselves, if we know we are a successful, vital and creative person, then lying around feels wrong and we will change that as quickly as possible. Our immune system is also linked to this when we treat ourselves well, eat, exercise, and enjoy life we tend to get fewer illnesses, so we get to feel good, look great and achieve amazing results. Are those people not the ones that make you feel good just being around?

Notes:

Get Ready, Get Set and Goal

Most things in life have a system, maybe a mathematical or logical one. Every machine has a system, a pattern followed to achieve the outcome it (and you) want. How annoying is it when you are preparing for a meeting or a holiday, packed and ready to go, and you load the car up, and when you turn the key... nothing happens! Dead, the silence screams at you, the usual pattern of the motor has not taken place so the outcome is not the one you wanted.

Setting goals or making a vision is personal, you can make them with other people business partner, spouse, child and you can help them as they can help you to stay on track, but you cannot do this for anyone else nor on their behalf.

Just to get you thinking about the types of people that do and don't set goals, you don't have to be a huge company like McDonalds or BP, nor do you have to be Sir Alex Ferguson or Sir Alan Sugar, but do you imagine for one second that they just got to be where they are in the world by just luck? Every day people are achieving things because they are planned and looking for opportunities, some people do get lucky and get to be successful at something but to keep it going needs goals and planning.

This is the key between the Lottery winners who fritter everything away and end up broke again and the ones that spend the rest of their lives financially free. That is probably the biggest dream or goal of most people, to be financially secure, knowing that all your bills are paid on time, your home secure and what you can then do for others. We all have dreams "what if", but there are many ways of winning the Lottery why keep it to just one!

Many people who set goals are seen as lucky and the strange thing is that the more you do it, the luckier you get. I love the part of my work where I get letters, or emails from people saying guess what.....I achieved or today I got. It is a system just like any other, it is not infallible, neither is the car engine. Putting all the components together they interlink and work. Just like the engine, it takes time and effort to keep it in good running order, commitment to goals is no different.

Write your goals down

There are thousands of books, DVDs, CDs, courses and now web pages that will validate the fact that writing down makes goals more definite. All our lives we are documented, birth, vaccines, school, college, work, marriage, bank, car, travel, & when we die. The certificates and records are there showing our progress, goals are the same. Writing them down also leaves an indelible mark on a page, to help us remember and also as a fantastic legacy to others.

What do you really want?

This is a BIGGY don't limit yourself or think of your Current Reality. Remove your limitations away, be really honest, remember you cannot fail, the only way not to succeed is to give up. Be honest with yourself, you need to take each individual goal and be clear, precise, amounts and quality. Saying I want to lose some weight...ok, one pound is some! I bet you do not really want to lose just one pound, or maybe get more money, one pound is also more money, again I bet you did not mean that. What did you mean, maybe twenty-eight pounds, or double your salary these are exact and you can monitor your progress, Not I want another car, what car, make model and year.

You will never be stimulated by a goal that is bland, insignificant or unclear paint a complete picture in your mind. Smells, textures, colours, the emotions you will be feeling when you have achieved it. Write it down as it makes it permanent.

Long and Short Term Goals

Once you have your goals identified, now it is time to break things down, you cannot eat an elephant in one go, but with bite-size pieces in time you can; your goals are the same.

Take responsibility for your goals; take action and ownership.

If you want to lose 28lbs you know logically you cannot do that healthily overnight or in two weeks (though we would like to) so, short-term goals for this one could be losing an average of one and a half pounds a week, so that would need eighteen weeks. Maybe have a nine week goal, to have reached the halfway mark of fourteen pounds, then a weekly goal for the weigh-in day. You need a short-term goal on a daily plan, maybe an eating or exercise guide. As you monitor your days and the weeks you keep track of your progress and your target, you may lose more and get to the goal of the fourteen pounds before the nine weeks, then you can adjust your long-term goal.

Remember goals are not in stone, you also need to plan through them so by the time you get to the halfway stage you will be looking at setting your new goal, once you have lost the 28lbs you may be looking at buying a special dress for your new figure, so the process starts again.

If your overall goal is to learn a new skill, like swimming. You can set a time frame and start lessons or get help from a friend to teach you. Break it down, once you have learnt to float and do a length of the pool you are swimming, so your goal then maybe to be able to swim 10 lengths of the pool, or even swim to raise money for charity.

So you are always building on your goals and achievements, you will see how absorbing and exciting this becomes.

Caring for the Caregiver

Procrastination and Congratulations

I like to bring this in here as many times it gets forgotten or left to last, procrastination is one of the biggest goal robbers, putting things off, finding excuses as to why it is not for me, or will not work for me. Guess what you will be right; if you do not do something different then nothing will change. I hear so often from people, I will start in the New Year, after my birthday, end of the tax year, after the wedding, on Monday, no doubt we have all been guilty of it at some time, but a saying from *Jim Rohn* a remarkable mentor *"for things to get better, I have to get better, for things to change, I have to change"* There is no doubt that these words are true.

How many times do you hear parents saying to children "if I have told you once, I have told you a thousand times" so why do they think that one thousand and one or one thousand and a hundred and one is going to make any difference? They need to be showing or telling the child in a different way, because that one is not working!

Start whatever it is you want to change today, right now, if something is not making you happy why wait to change it?

On the other side of the same coin when you have started your change procedure be kind to yourself, congratulate yourself, celebrate your achievements, even the ones you see as small, because they will lead you on to bigger ones. Celebrating your achievement of losing the 1st pound is as important as the 28th pound, because without losing the first one you would never have achieved the other one.

Write your congratulations on your goal sheet, stick on stars or big ticks, have you seen the beaming smile of a child coming home from school with the well done or gold star on their work, they feel like they can take on the world. As adults we are no different, encouragement and praise are good for us too. Do remember our goals are for us, so if we are waiting for praise and congratulations from other people, we may be waiting a long time. So don't be shy, pat yourself on the back, treat yourself to something nice and say well done me. You will then be more enthused to achieve your next goal on the ladder.

Don't Make Your Goals too Easy

The idea of setting goals is to achieve something you really want; breaking them into short-term goals gives you the stepping stones along the way. If you do not challenge yourself you will not change and grow, but don't set yourself up to give up either.

If your long-term goal is to walk a tightrope between two skyscrapers, then you would not even attempt that without many short-term goals along the way, not only to learn to walk on a tightrope and balance, your health and fitness would need work, so don't be too narrow in your goal setting.

Challenge yourself and learn, then move your goal to the next one. Each part should be a pleasure, we do not goal set to demand or make ourselves feel bad this is an evolutionary process that makes us better at anything that we want to achieve.

No Rose Coloured Glasses

Don't think that what you are taking on here is not a challenge, because it is. If it were that easy everyone would be doing it, just the same as making 1,000,000 Dollars, Pounds or Euros it is possible but not everyone does it.

Nor do you expect everything and every day to be perfect, because life is just not like that. See obstacles or difficult situation on the horizon, see them, accept them and plan for them. When I am mentoring especially for weight loss very often I hear "I had a bad day, because I overlaid and did not take my lunch with me, so the day was ruined", when you set your goals to have some suitable something either in the fridge at work, or in your desk drawer. Rather than going to the chip shop or grabbing a sandwich, pop to a local shop and get a cooked piece of chicken or lean meat.

When you go out with friends and you don't want to drink, but they are insisting and you feel that your determination is not yet strong enough carry a small tube of toothpaste in your bag, pop to the loo and rub some on your teeth, wine and alcohol taste horrible, so it will help you stay strong and then you can make your own choices.

There is no doubt that "things" will come along and trip us up along the route to change, but it is not a disaster just a hiccup. Maybe learn from it and adjust your short-term goals so that if the situation arises again you will be prepared. Don't be hard on yourself or give up, nothing worth achieving was gained without surmounting a few molehills along the way.....just don't let them turn into mountains.

This is also where your WHY is so important, if you really want something and see yourself with it, nothing will deter you. You will turn into a person on a mission, full speed ahead until you reach the target.

Your Progress

Tracking what you are doing is important, when you write things down you can then tick them off as they are achieved Giving you a visual achievement sheet: remember the gold stars and the self-congratulations? A much better way to change than under threat - there will be a lot less resistance to your new future.

Two reasons for change Please or Pain, moving towards pleasure or away from pain, whichever is your motive start by highlighting your achievements. pleasure will take over. A secondary consequence of change, is the effect on other people, you may become a threat to others as they are not ready to change, sometimes you leave people, places and things behind, even if they are trying to keep you. Think about anyone who travels or joins the forces, they have to go away from their home, family and friends. They come back, but not as the same person, they have changed and grown by the choices and experiences they have had.

Have you ever been to a school or work reunion? People that were friends or even close friends at that time now are like strangers, because your lives have taken different paths. It may be good to catch up, and a new relationship may emerge but it is not the same as the old one.

My favourite one of these is always a previous girlfriend or boyfriend, you can be madly in love in your younger years and bitterly heartbroken at the ending of the relationship, when you see them or bump into them years later, most of the time the reaction is, whatever did I see in them! Because we have moved on and grown up in our own lives.

Your progress will incur changes to people around you, it is up to them if they enhance it or try to hinder it, and it is up to you to keep to your goals and your new future.

Don't Do This Alone

As I have said from the start of this book, nobody has achieved their goals all by themselves, whatever we want to achieve people have gone before us that we can learn from. Find as much support and like-minded people as you can, join clubs, societies or classes, anything that is related to what you want to achieve. Learn from the Masters and learn from their mistakes. Every successful person will tell you about how they achieved their goals and share their struggles along the way.

If you want to write professionally, join clubs either locally or on the net, talk to published people, ask questions and listen to talks and seminars, be a sponge for information to help you along. If you want to write but surround yourself with bricklayers you are not going to absorb or learn the right skills. If you want to be a bricklayer then you do not want to be

Surrounding yourself with people and information on internet marketing. I hope you see the point here, no matter what you want there is information and there are people out there to help and advise you. Take full advantage of all of it, then it is very likely you will miss some of the rocks in the road to your new destination.

Talking to people about what you want is very important too, I have found a lot of people starting up in business don't want to tell their spouses or their family, a business without advertising is not going to grow. The more people you tell the more likely it is you will get a client, the more people you tell about your goals the more likely you are to get to know people in that particular area.

We talked earlier about positive and negative people, you will come across both, choose who you want to spend time and energy with. Never assume people will not be interested, or will not listen to you, if you believe in you and what you want then the passion is infectious and you never know who or what they know that can help you.

Also, when you talk to people and share your goals, when the rocks in the road or the obstacle jump out at you another viewpoint can make them look a lot smaller, often giving you another way to get around them.

Gratitude

It is important, no matter what your Current Reality is right now, no matter how bad you think it is, there is always something to be grateful for. Having each new day, to have the opportunity to change for the future. Once you stop looking at all the things you do not have, you can channel your thoughts to a future of what you do want. You Current Reality is not forever,

Be thankful for the people who are in your life, they might not be the ones that you want to be there in the future, but they are part of the reason you want to change, you have learnt something from every single one of them.

Be thankful for all the lessons that you have learnt to bring you to the point that you know that the future can be different if you want it to be.

Caring for the Caregiver

The Missing Links

Ok, having put these into place there are still three missing links, Affirmations, Visualisation and Action.

Caring for the Caregiver

Affirmations

Once you have your goals, you need to write them in a way that they are stimulants for you, to affirm your goals into a lifelike experience. So every affirmation must be owned, so it is written in the 1st person I, Me, Myself. They are also written in the present tense, in the here and now. There is no hopes, wishes, dreams, maybes, ifs, coulds, shoulds, or woulds.

Example:
I wish I had more money and a better job. This will not paint any positive picture of change.

I am happy and thankful that all of my bills are paid on time and there is extra money in the bank from my salary as the Marketing Manager

I am thrilled now that I travel to the conference in New York first class as the new Marketing Manager

For each goal write an affirmation, there is no exact guaranteed format, but positive, active, outcomes in one sentence is what you need.

Visualisation

I said earlier about setting your goals with as many details as possible, in this internet age this becomes really exciting, I used to say to people build a picture board or scrapbook that you can keep in a handy place and look at regularly to reinforce your goals. But with free online pictures and imagines it is easy to build up a mini-movie, personal to your own goals, this is something that you can even put to music and have captions to enhance the visualisation process.

Put together your own future in pictures and words, sit quietly and watch it through several times a day. With the written affirmations you need to sit quietly and read each one through, close your eyes and imagine the scene. So you can visualise your new reality, building the new picture up in your mind which will be imposed into your sub conscious mind. The picture board is always a good option as well.

Action

It is no good wishing for change, with your affirmations taking time to visualise the new you, or your new reality is still in the realms of wishful thinking, though as the pictures get internalised and get stronger your behaviour will automatically change to achieve the outcomes you want.

Choosing to change your behaviour and your actions will help and enhance the process, remember what I said about talking to people, going to classes, seminars, looking for information, this is action you are turning your behaviour towards your outcomes.

If you want to change shape and lose weight, then changing your shopping choices, joining a gym or buying an exercise DVD are all actions towards your new reality.

Make sure your actions progress each day, that way you are then behaving like the person you want to be. Go test drive the car you want, go view the houses until you find the one that fits your requirements. Go to join dance classes or a speaking group, all of which will help your progression, skills and achievements towards your goal.

Notes:

Last but Not Least

I bet the question on your lips is How long will it take? Well, there is no magic wand, if you have set your goals and broken them down into small steps, you may well have set a timescale for that, you may achieve the short-term goals sooner or later than expected so you can adjust your overall goal.

A goal has no expiry date it is valid until you no longer want it or you achieve it. It is never too late to start, or too hard to try. The only limits are the ones you accept. That is why there are people of seventy or eighty years of age wing walking or skydiving, they are getting married, moving countries and running in marathons.

There are no ends to the possibilities of what you could want, just because it is not what is right for others does not make it wrong. Winston Churchill was not Prime Minister until after normal retirement age; Charlotte Church was an international singing star at the age of twelve, before Roger Bannister ran a four minute mile it was thought to be impossible, that record has been well and truly smashed.

Something is only impossible until it has been done, then it is a target that somebody will want to improve on.

Your goals should be never ending, as they will grow and develop with you. As you get towards one you set the next, the excitement and your capabilities only get bigger and better. Do you remember what I said earlier about being lucky and how successful people are luckier, then you will see you will also be one of the "luckiest" people around.

Caring for the Caregiver

CHAPTER 6

As I think, say and believe…I am

Affirmations are to affirm the way we want our new current reality to be, visualisations are to visualise the way we want to see our new current reality, action is to make our behaviour correct for our personal living in our new current reality.

If we can conceive it, believe it, we can create it. At the unveiling of the Epcot Centre the Centre Director in his opening speech said "if only Walt could have seen it", Walt Disney, the mind behind it had died before the completion of the Centre, but his widow was there to represent him and in reply she told the audience that "Walt had seen it, he had seen it long before anyone else".

Athletes have used these visualisation techniques for many years, golfers, archers, all know where their ball or arrow is going to end up before they hit or release them. They visualise the target and through many repetitions of taking the shot they know the tension and force needed in their muscles, it becomes almost automatic.

Keeping positive self-talk flowing enhances your abilities to be as good as you can be, instead of dipping under stress and self-doubt. Believe in yourself, your worth, your efficacy and your abilities to deserve whatever it is that you really want. Talk to yourself positively, be your own best friend, encourage, support and praise yourself.

One of the most magical men I have heard, way before all this self-development and goal setting, or understanding of how the mind and human brain functions, like we now do, was Mohamed Ali. At the time he was thought big headed, vain, sometimes even ridiculous, but what a man! He instinctively knew about the power of his mind, the power of belief and the importance of self-talk. He made up rhymes about himself his strength, his power, his ability and about his opponent's weaknesses. He would sing them repeatedly reaffirming them in his mind. You don't have to be in the situation physically, but when your visualization's vividness are strong enough your mind sees them as reality.

If he had gone into the ring against the giants of men that he fought thinking, ohhh maybe I can hit him, or ok if it gets too bad I can lie down on the canvas. He would never have been World Champion in the first place, then to come back and do it over again, not once but twice, this man's mind was even stronger than his body. That is what got him through and took him to the very top.

Another person who has taken the world by storm but not in a rip-roaring way is Susan Boyle, she had a dream for so many years, through very turbulent years of growing up, so many people not believing that she was capable. She put into action a plan to get to the audition and sing. She took three buses and arrived hours before the auditions, people did not even think that she could get herself to the audition, but she did.

However, she had got to a previous audition and seeing the crowds, gave into her own doubts and went home again. She still believed in herself, did not give up and went back again, walked out on the stage, even then she was getting disrespectful looks, people were judging her, but once she opened her mouth and started to sing.

The rest as we say is history!

These type of people are important to all of us, some people achieve goals early, then they have to set new ones and achieve them again, others may wait a long time to achieve, but as I said in the section about time limits all the while the goal is important to you then you can still achieve it.

Some Will, Some Won't, So What?

I was introduced to this phrase many years ago in a marketing seminar, and I was quite taken back by it, because I did care about the "so what", I spent many years self-examining about what I had done wrong, or what could I have done differently to make the difference. After many exhausting self-interrogations and attending hundreds of hours of courses, seminars, conferences and bring up a feisty teenager I finally realised that it does not matter that I care, if they don't.

So, just like all of the people reading this book, some will follow it to the letter and write out their goals, examine their self-talk, practice the affirmations and take time to invest in themselves, just like there will be people that won't. So what does that mean? That now is the right time for some and not for others, not just because of my book, but because of where your lives are at the moment. I believe that self-development is like opening a safe to find an onion inside.

None of us, who have developed or trained or achieved anything have only done it once, we have had various inputs and information, just like the lock on a safe each piece of information that comes along that is right for us, at the time we receive it is a click on the dial, after four or five of those clicks we get more interested and want to know more, find out more and put into practice things we are finding out. As the safe door opens we find the onion inside, then we are looking at the layers of the onion that we peel back in ourselves to then go on in a new way. This process can take a longer or shorter time, the number of layers we peel back is up to us.

It is also important to remember that people around us may not be in the same stage of change that we are, so it is up to them how or when they change or not as the case may be.

This is not a deeply psychological book, nor is it spiritual, nor medical we may never truly know or understand how this process works, but there again maybe we do not need to. Perhaps the outcomes will outweigh the unknown, or maybe we will want to take our knowledge to a deeper depth on one or several of the options. That is a choice we make. The one thing I hope everyone can take from this book is that we are responsible for our self, we have choices and we have free will, once we accept the responsibility, acceptance and accountability for our self, then there really is nothing that we cannot do, be or have. We can design, make and live our world just as we want it.

The Show Must Go On

If you have ever been involved in amateur dramatics, public speaking, teaching, demonstrating etc. you will know the importance of rehearsals, how many times do you try something before it is right; then even on the night, if it is live, there are still a lot of things that can go wrong. Of course, if you are filming or recording something, you can always edit out the mistakes. Your visualising and affirmations are just like this.

The way to build your new picture into your subconscious mind is to go over and over it, rehearse it until you know it inside out until the picture is clear and precise. Role play in your mind anything that you can anticipate that will be a rock in your road, overcome the obstacle and carry on your journey.

If you were doing your first amateur play, and you rehearsed your lines, knew all your cues, your costume perfect; then on the night the lights did not work, you would be in a flap and upset, but because you are in a production there are other people around you that have done many performances, they have been through many hitches; so their experience and assurance is needed to help you through, the technicians are there to change a fuse and the lights all come on again.....So the show goes on and you deliver beautifully, you are proud of yourself and your performance. There is always a need of good support.

In a few years, when you have done many performances, glided through many hitches and reassured many up and coming starlet you look back at the home video of that first performance and shudder, because you have come such a long way. You have improved in confidence, timing, style, presentation, voice, diction, poise and so much more. This is because as you progress you develop more and more until you become the best you can be, then onto a new goal. Many actors go from being at the top of their field in comedy acting, and then they want to do thrillers or classics and round the other way of course. This is the concept of development; all the while you are learning and growing, by challenging yourself.

The old saying of practice makes perfect, well we are not perfect but rehearsing your future in your mind if a great way or knowing exactly how it will feel, what you will be like, how you will live, so these written two-dimensional goals are now three-dimensional, or even a hologram of your future.

As you rehearse your future and then come back to current reality, you will find the strength, power, energy and resources to achieve your new future. You will also attract to you the people that are right for that new future.

Maximising the Visualising; Affirmation Process

If you were going to build your own house, you would not just walk up to any old piece of land and lay a few bricks with superglue, or knock some nails in a piece of wood with the heel of a shoe; you would plan where you wanted to be and what type of house you wanted; draw many rough sketches of the outside and of each room, rub out and add many ideas before the architect or surveyor even got involved; prepare plans, licences, permissions, plant and machinery, materials and a workforce; collect information about local services and amenities. Then as the work progressed you would be there each and every day to oversee your project as your dream becomes a reality.

When you are going to build your own future, you also need adequate, efficient and correct tools to do the job. Beliefs, self-talk, self-esteem, self-efficacy, comfort zones, goals, affirmations, and visualization are the tools to make the blueprint for the life that you want to live; all you have to do, is go and live it.

Each affirmation is important to you, not cutting corners or skipping a few, you are a product of your investment.

1. I said in the previous chapter that affirmations must be in the 1st Person, me, myself, and I. This is not selfish or egoistic, it is a fact that you can only change YOU, not anyone else and not for somebody else. If you try do make affirmations for somebody else they will fail, sorry to be so blunt but maybe you can spend that time on your affirmations for yourself.

You need to see yourself, living, behaving, enjoying and succeeding in the way you want to be. If at first, you have difficulties seeing yourself in the long-term goal, the short-term goals come into play, as you achieve them you will be able to visualise yourself towards your long-term goal.

Writing your affirmations in the 1st person makes you take responsibility for the action and outcome, no loopholes to blame others, skills or circumstances

2. The other thing that was stated in the previous chapter was in the Present Tense, the here and now

The reason affirmations are written in the present tense is because you want to see yourself as already having achieved the goal. This is the picture you are going to put into your subconscious so when the picture is so strong and it clashes with your current reality....zoom you get super-charged to move towards the new picture.

Write affirmations for your short-term goals as well, remember the stepping stones over the river you need each and every single one to get to the other side in the best condition, to take the best advantage of all the new opportunities the other side has to offer.

Are you still sceptical, are you thinking that this is all a lie! Have there not been any lights going on or arrhh ha moments up to now?

It is not a lie, nor is it a magic wand, remember Gestalt and moving the picture until you feel comfortable, you are moving the picture in your mind to go straight to where you want and how you want it to be. With your affirmations you are giving sanction to a new picture of how you see things, you are strengthening your own resolve to say that your current reality in that particular area of your life needs to change to be your future reality.

Also remember NO shoulds, coulds, woulds, if, or maybes but also no skill words like try, intend to, attempt, will see. These are loopholes and you are not going to let yourself squirm out of a hole and blame others!

We can't live in the past no matter how great or awful it was, time waits for no man or woman come to that. The present is fleeting we can only build for the future.

I am not devaluing memories here, nor am I saying we cannot and do not learn from the past and present but we cannot healthily live in a time warp of the past.

Good Practice Guide

Affirmations are positive, bright, happy enjoyable and short. We are not going to read a ten-page affirmation, so concise and punchy is always great.

All affirmations are about what you want and not about what you don't want or what you want to change. Also, remember that words trigger pictures for us, so be careful what you paint.

I have talked throughout the book about the need to make your affirmations clear, precise and detailed add, emotions, smells and textures, as the more real you make your affirmations the stronger the picture will be. If you know exactly what you want, it will make finding it so much easier. You would not go to an Indian restaurant and order Italian food, nor would you expect the waiter to order for you as you are not sure what you want, you may ask for suggestions but finally you would make the choice.

Don't compete or compare in your affirmations, nobody is the same as you and you are not the same as anyone else, you do not need bigger, better, smaller, thinner than. You want what is right for you. You will meet people that have more experience than you, have achieved more than you and you should learn from them, you will also meet people who know less and have achieved less than you, these people you should help with your knowledge and know how.

None of us are born experts, we learn and choose what we want to know, neither is there one single person who is an expert in everything. You need to have a balance in your life so remember to affirm in a wide array of areas of your life. As humans, we are better balanced and focused that way we can move forward most effectively.

Visualisation is not always easy for everyone, some people find it hard to quieten their mind, so maybe calming music, or even silence for a while before you sit comfortably to visualise, you can make a recording of you talking your affirmations through, remember learning to ride a bike, the more you do it the easier it gets. Keep at it and don't give up. You are worth the effort.

Affirmations also help us to keep our word to ourselves, remember way back in the book when we thought about how we treat ourselves; we need to learn that a promise to our self is as important as a promise to anyone else. Also, it helps in the way we speak to ourselves as affirmations are positive, happy and enjoyable, so our self-talk is enhanced and makes us feel good about ourselves.

Sometimes it will seem like a ping-pong match in your head about your old self and your new self, but as soon as the new vision becomes stronger that will stop.

Suggestions for Affirmations

I am a happy and successful person, I am open to change and enjoy new challenges. I am happy and content living in my new home, I am thankful for all the help I receive, I love spending quality time with my children, I speak well in public, I respect myself and people around me.
I see all challenges as opportunities.
I enjoy my life & all the loving relationships that surround me.
I care about my health and I am worth looking after.
I take pride in myself and everything I do.
I encourage people around me to be the best they can be.
I enjoy each day as a new adventure and make the most of each opportunity.
I am thrilled with my new shape body, I love being able to exercise and feel my toned muscles, I enjoy eating fresh, healthy food.

Now You:

Let's Get To Work

Once you have your long and short-term goals identified and determined, got your progress strategy organised, got your affirmations written out, then it is time to get to work.

Then the fun begins. Go through your affirmations twice a day, I like first thing in the morning to start my day in a positive way and last thing at night to end the day in a positive way. There is an important clause here it is never a chore or a bore; remember you choose to do this you don't have to.

It does not take long just seconds to a minute an affirmation, depending on the content, but this is already changing your attitude to yourself and how important your own development is. I usually spend about 30mins on my affirmations, does not matter when you do this but quiet and concentration is a must.

Read, Picture and Feel, each affirmation, in turn, I prefer to close my eyes when I visualise, I bring in as much detail, taste, touch, smell and emotion as possible. You play the picture just as you would see the scene as if you are there in everyday life, you don't need to look at the scene with you in it because emotion then is very hard to do.

Then the magic key, do it again and again and again each and every day it does take time to imprint into our minds, so just keep going and enjoy every second of every time you do it. There is always one BUT, don't get into the habit of thinking all goals take a long time to achieve, you may just be surprised at how quickly change comes when you are ready, willing and open to new adventures.

Have fun; the world is now yours for the taking, I always like to hear about your achievements and outcomes, so there is always an open invitation to anyone reading this book to send me their experiences and outcomes directly to my website. www.lindasage.com I have used some of my own experiences and those of others throughout the book not in a way to say look what we can do or what we have achieved, but to show you that we all start from somewhere and we are all capable of making the future that we want for ourselves.

So, now just go and design yours.

Six Years On

Caring for the Caregiver

Chapter 7 - Six Years On

Six years on..... Where does time go? Well, I must have been having fun for it to fly by in a blink of an eye. This is something I hear from so many people, where has the day gone, the week, the month, the year, and decades. One concept is sure, if we are lucky we have more time; but there are many that have not had as much as they thought.

There is no exact science of life, nor is there any guarantee or infinite span allotted to us, what I have learnt more than anything is to appreciate and value each minute, don't wish them away, or pass on enjoying them; each one is unique and never to be repeated. Life is not fair at times, but it is equal no matter where you are on the planet, you all have the same twenty-four hours in each and every day. Everything else can be bought or replaced; time does not offer that luxury. This is one lesson that has really been learnt in these ensuing years. The other is that success, achieving goals or dreams, whichever term you prefer, is a purely personal experience, one you can share with others, but even then it is different for all involved. The planet, life, the universe will never run out of possibilities, in fact the more successful people are the more opportunities, inventions, books, apps, cars, whatever you can think of, because whenever something has been created from an idea, somebody else will come along and want to improve on it.

It does not matter what you see as success, as long as it matters to you. Most people aim for financial security, their own business, their dream, house, boat, clothes or jewels. In all of the decades, the dreams have been the same. Some people have reached them, some more will reach them, but some will not, and that is not because they do not have the potential, or the possibility, but because they did not follow it and hang onto it.

I would like you for a moment think of what you have achieved in the last day, week, month or year. Learning to do and maintaining a reflective log, makes looking back so much easier and you do not forget the smaller goals along the way. The three main words, for me to help people move forward are determination, perseverance and resilience, as well as being personally responsible and accountable. With these traits you cannot lose, you have to move forward and all the while you are moving change will happen. Lots of people say it is luck, but without asking for what you want and working towards it, you will not be able to achieve it.

When I was very young before I knew all about psychology or mindset, my mum took me to the cinema to see Born Free, a magic happened for me and a lifetime affection for felines was born. The planes and views of South Africa were indelibly etched into my mind. It was on my "To Do" list for over five decades, before I got there and I was not disappointed. The scenery, the people, the food, the amazing sunsets and the multi-colour nation were amazing, the helicopter ride over the peninsular, the white sand beaches, diving in a cage with sharks, the Capes and wildlife roaming around were as I had imagined. However, the safari with the big five 4 ticked the boxes, the majesty of the elephants, the elegance of the giraffes, the vitality of the zebras were breathtaking, but my icing on my cake with a huge cherry on the top was seeing the lions in their habitat. One lion surrounded by his three lionesses, pure magic, well worth waiting every minute to see that and something I will never forget.

Sometimes we have to be more patient, but worth the wait, others come to fruition in super quick time, when you prioritize and aim for them.

One area I would like to bring in here, very often we hold on to hopes, dreams, belongings and people too long. As we move forward and change, our environments change and so do our circle of people, some will be there for longer or shorter periods, but there is something to learn from all of them, especially the ones who hurt us and try to derail us. We learn much more about ourselves in the trying times, than in the calmer times. Challenges and change come hand in hand.

I did mention earlier in the book about my dream house in Spain, at one time I was concentrating so hard to accomplish this goal, I was knocked for six when it literally split and trying to sort it out was a huge nightmare, the bank nor the insurance company were any use. In fact, the bank putting so much pressure on me, was what made me hold up my hands and say, I need to give up on this one and move on. When I moved into that house I was convinced I would be leaving it in a box, that was me for the rest of my life.

I not only got screwed financially by the banks, but my husband's business partner and my business associates all in the space of eighteen months, that's is on top of the previous eighteen months with losing both parents and ex-husband, as well as my daughter running into as many disasters possible. I was financially, emotionally and mentally in pieces.

When opportunity came knocking in the form of the Middle East, the offer to work there was another soul saver. Not an easy country to be in, and the environment was challenging on all fronts, but I met some incredible people, had new opportunities and was able to cut my ties to my previous dream. By being away, I was able to return and see that the house was no longer a dream I needed, in fact, it had become a dream that was dragging me down and stopping me moving forward. Sorting out the house everyone's belongings and downsizing was the only option, but it was not a sad option. My reality had changed.

In fact, over the next few years, the dream of the big house, with its own pool and extensive land has become a complete void. A nice comfortable place with easy access, no garden responsibilities, easily cleaned (can't tell you how many hours I have spent cleaning and gardening in my life.) Now happiness is, small utility bills, compact living with items that mean something special to me. Off-loading rubbish and excess, belongings that before I saw as needs; now get relegated to boot sales or charity shops. All those kitchen gadgets and must-haves are mere memories; practicality and usefulness now define my needs. That is not to say that in a few years, what I see now as totally necessary will be not be following its predecessors.

Learning to appreciate the here and now is a big lesson to learn, and one, unfortunately, that seems to take us a long time, usually well into adulthood and beyond.

Finding a way to keep yourself on track is vitally important, not just personal accountability, my best advice and my greatest time of self-growth and achievement have always come when I am working with a mentor. Somebody at least two rungs up the ladder above where you are, and where you want to be. Many say it is an expense, but it really is not; it is an investment in you and your future. It will also stop you making costly mistakes, as they will always share their potholes and mishaps with you. Learn from their mistakes and it will save you, even more time, in getting the success you want.

You have to be focused, be willing to work the extra time, go the extra mile and know that the journey is as important as the achieving of the goal.

Learning to live and love yourself, it is true that unless you know you, how can you give to somebody else. There is a song Cher sings, "At some time we all sleep alone." my mum said this to me a long time before the song came out and it did not resonate with me till many years later.

Asking for what you want is also an important lesson, I am not saying demanding or bullying, but talking to people, share your vision and be open about the help you need. When you are looking for something you will find it, others have a wealth of experience and knowledge; it might just be what you need. Remember in no type of relationship can you or others read minds, openness, clarity and sharing get much better results; than struggling on alone.

I have had some amazing mentors in my time, people who have seen traits and possibilities in me, that I never knew existed. Even now, my latest mentors are all younger than me, you may think "What can they teach me?" Let me tell you, a lot; the world is changing and like it or not we have to change with it. My techno knowledge and abilities have improved, but some people have been very patient and understanding with me. Also, all the while I am learning and having difficulties grasping what they are teaching me, it makes me aware of how my mentees and attendees feel with the knowledge that I am comfortable with.

Going back through my original book Personal Coaching for Change, all the sections still hold very true, we have not changed the way in which we think, or behave from our beliefs. Nor does anyone really want to achieve anything was not wanted then, but tools and global access have made it easier, more effective in the way we can command change and achievement

However, there are golden keys that I would like to highlight in this section and as we say hindsight is great, but now we can see where we made mistakes in the past and we can do something about them for the future.

My top 20 Must Do, or Must Have for Success

1. Know what you want; finding your passion, your direction, what you see as success, is your starting point. Without a fixed reference point, working towards it is very difficult. That is not to say, that once you are on your way and achieving the interim goals, your end goal will not change, move or get bigger. That is fine, but don't keep changing the endpoint before you start, or you will never start.

2. Break it down into smaller measurable achievements, and write it all down, then daily goals each one a step towards where you want to be. You may have different areas that you need to work on to attain your ultimate success, so write a daily goal to achieve in each area. Your big goal may be well out there, far beyond your belief system at the moment, that is fine; remember you don't need to know the how; just a powerful why. The journey to success will not usually be on the shortest route, to smaller goals and measurable outcomes will keep you moving towards your target.

3. Persistence: so many people in this fast set world, want instant results, magic solutions, that are not viable or sustainable. Keep at it. Just a few small deeds, or steps on a daily basis will get you where you want to be, plus it forms good practice habits, that will always be helpful.

4. Accountability: Tell people, about what you are doing, document your journey the good and the bad, it will help others who follow you. Ask somebody to make you demonstrate your progress and achievements.

5. Be teachable: get a mentor, someone who is where you want to be, somebody who has your interest at heart and will help you save, money time and heartache. Be a sponge and act upon what you learn.

6. Personal integrity: Keep your word to yourself, value your needs, your work and your achievements. When you set goals, achieve them, be the person that others want to do business with, want to ask for help, want to be your best.

7. Ask for what you want, share your needs and your weaknesses, let others help you and find solutions for you. If you have a talent, a gift, an invention or a service that can help others, why do you not want to tell them? Keeping it to yourself does nobody any favours.

8. Cut off your opt-outs, burning bridges, close doors and move forward. All the time you know there is a way to retreat, whenever the going gets tough you will go running back to the safe and secure area. Stand your ground, stabilize yourself and then progress. We all have wobbles and insecurities at times, it does not mean it is time to give up and throw in the towel.

9. Let go of dead wood: We all like the familiar and the security blankets that we have around us. But, if they are no longer useful, let them go; whether they are belongings, people, places, habits, or beliefs. There is an old saying "If you are not part of the solution, you are part of the problem." This is very true in your progress, ties holding you back will need to be broken, but if you are letting them hold you back, and not proactively cutting them, you will never move forward. Don't be afraid to let go there are plenty more of everything to replace them.

10. Resilient: Be like Teflon, let the past slide, let people go who are not moving forward with you (remember that is their choice, you can only drag them so far, kicking and screaming.) Don't believe the negative wizards out there, as they will always be there. Life and challenges do not always go to plan, but believing in yourself, your abilities and your success are paramount, picking yourself up, dusting off and putting the next foot forward.

11. Ban excuses: You can have progress or you have excuses, you can't have both. Procrastination is the biggest thief, of time, goals, achievements and the biggest cause of regret, guilt and blame. You can think of a thousand excuses as to why not to achieve, or move forward, but there is not a single reason; know and understand the difference. (Accountability helps with this).

12. Be consistent: It creates expectancy. If you are able to allocate a certain time, or certain budget to your goals at this time, that is fine. Keep to it no matter what. Think about your life, you like consistency, when you turn the shower on you expect hot water, because it is usually there. When you put the key in the car, you expect it to start; you have built your plans around the expected consistency. When it is not there, you get frustrated and upset. So, just the same with life, business and achieving goals, be consistent in your progress and you will come to expect better outcomes, more achievements and your clients will come to think of you for their consistency, for your success will be assured.

13. Reflect: Reflection is hugely important, learn from your mistakes and see what is working well. Why are you pouring money, time and effort into something that is not helping you move forward? Regular reflection, build it into your day, your week, or your project plan. It will save you time, money and effort in the long run.

14. Break out of your comfort zones: A long time I was told, "You only start learning and changing at the outside edge of your comfort zone." Very true, expanding and reforming comfort zones is hugely important; after all fears and phobias are only very restrictive comfort zones, once they have a bigger stretch the less scary old constraints feel.

15. Celebrate: each and every achievement celebrate it, because without it you will not move onto the next one. If I am mentoring in business I always suggest that 10% of each sale goes into a celebration fund. So the first one, is a small but none the less important celebration, if the next goal is ten, the celebration is 10 times as big, etc. etc. Even with weight loss and personal achievements, you can set up a pot of weekly achievements, so that once you hit the milestones, you can treat yourself well.

16. Treat yourself well: This is probably one of the biggest ones, treat yourself well not just regulating your self-talk, but treating your body, health and overall wellbeing as a priority. In business, if you are not at the top of your game, your business will not be either, if you want to climb the career ladder; leading by example is key; if you want a great relationship, looking the best you can and feeling great is important. So, eat well, sleep well, hydrate well, exercise and make time in your schedule for MeX, whatever it is you like doing, do it. Relax, refuel and revitalize. This time is as important as any meeting or project, without it over time the rest will collapse.

17. Choose your attitude: Just think of the people who make you happy, make you laugh and listen to you. Join them and be a person that people want around, be interested in others and open to new adventures, new opportunities. Your attitude will determine your altitude. Your choice how high you want to fly.

18. Choose happiness: It is a choice, sometimes you do not think so, but there is always a choice and as we have life, it surely is better to make the most of it. Laughter is a huge stimulant, a wonderful medicine and stimulates endorphins that counteract free radicals that go hand in hand with worry, stress and poor health.

19. Learn to speak in public: You may think this is a little strange, but in all areas of life if you can speak confidently, competently and precisely, putting your thoughts, ideas, business across well; you are light years ahead of your competition. Whether it is socially, for an interview, or professionally. It does not have to cost a fortune, there are several organizations, I was greatly helped by Toastmasters International, there will always be a group near you, or now they are online too.

20. Be sincere: To yourself and to others, knowing what you want and your why are very personal; don't copy others because you will uncomfortable and others will feel uncomfortable with you. You are unique and can bring something to the table nobody else can. Find your style, your way of doing tasks, your way of progressing. After all, this is working for your success, not for the success as a copy of! Many people will forgive many mistakes, but being false is the biggest way of turning people away from you. Feel at peace with you and who you are, others will either accept it or not, but that is their choice.

A Letter to Self:

Whether you are of a generation that lived through a war, or have any contacts with a military background, I think that you may know what a "Dear John" letter is. But, just in case; it was a term used in World War 2 and has diversified into many areas now of a letter or text in more modern days, telling the recipient that a relationship is over, that the writer has moved on and usually found somebody else, who they felt more close to and loved profoundly.

I want you to take this concept and imagine if your dreams, hopes and goals wrote a "Dear John" letter to you. If they gave up on you and walked away.

Dear (Your name) Linda,
It is with deep regret and sadness that I feel the need to write to you and tell you it is time I moved on. I have been patient and forgiving, I have waited in line for your attention, you very often made me promises and then continually broke them. Very often you put others before me; you gave in and just left me hanging.

Many years have passed, many people come and gone, but I was always here for you, excited you, developed you and gave you hope when others let you down, but it seems it was not enough.

I feel bruised, abused and battered, just taken off of the shelf, dusted off and ignited when you felt like it, to then be deflated and abandoned on many, many occasions. Though, I want you to know that I really enjoyed a lot of our time together, the learning and the enthusiasm, the passion and the desire we shared will always remain with me as comforting memories.

Your endless "To Do" lists, vision boards, and diaries always spurred me on to believe there was still a flame burning for me. The money you spent on the Self-Help, How To books and courses, all kept me bouncing and hoping. Then each time my emotions would be dashed and hurt. There were times when you were proactively chasing me, such delight, and exhilaration, but unfortunately as time as has gone on those times got further and further apart and with less intensity.

You got out of being "us" and back into being you. Choosing new companions, apathy and procrastination, who robbed me of your company and your attention. I shed many tears waiting for you to come back to me, but now I have to make the decision for my future, for my life and for my dreams. I still have them, I still want to enjoy them, but alas I am now convinced that they will not be with you.

I am moving on, to somebody who can care and nourish me, will pay me attention and develop me into something bigger and better. Will let me grow and enjoy all our time together, somebody who can see and appreciate my benefits and my tenacity, somebody who is able and willing to go that extra mile to understand my needs and my complexities to achieve success together by living the successful life that you have given up on.

(Your name) Linda, I am truly sorry that it has come to this, but you have changed and surround yourself with feelings that suffocate and stifle me. Negativity seems to be blocking your vision and lethargy seems to keep you stationary. I am sorry, but that is an environment that I cannot survive in.

I wish you all the very best in your life with your new companions, and I hope they will make you happy, as I did not quite get the chance to change your world.

Take care of yourself.

Your loving friends
    Dreams, Hopes and Goals.

Is this a letter that you would really like to receive? Just like all the recipients of "Dear John" letters sadness and regret hit you, so to stop this happening, before your treasured dreams, hopes and goals become mere memories, it is time for action and time to be proactive.

Make each day count and win them all back, enjoy them and live your success with them banishing all the negative creatures from your mind and your actions.

There is still time to cement your relationship and make a difference.

The graveyards all around the world are full of magnificent inventions, marvelous books and outstanding achievements, all because they left it too late and time run out. As I said at the start of this section, time is our greatest asset; we have to make the most of it.

I have been very lucky and lived many decades, and hope there are many more exciting ones to come, but in reality……. Who knows?

Be kind to yourself, be supportive and thoughtful of others, but value all of you equally, your dreams, hopes, goals are no less worthy than anyone else. Don't relinquish your passion, find a way to make it happen and be happy.

Many years ago, people went into a job at 16 and had the expectancy of a job for life, the world is not like that anymore, the internet and the ease of travel make anything possible. Even the smallest business, has a worldwide marketplace, so whatever it is you want, you can find it; support, knowledge, information, a spouse, a house, a car, a product or a service. This was somebody else's dream to provide it, their dream came true with hard work and persistence. Make yours come true too.

You have the potential, you have the ability and you have the accessibility of all the tools, know-how and support you need. Go for it, make the most of it and when you reflect back on your life, there will be no regrets, no what ifs, just a wonderful adventure and amazing stories to tell about your achievements and conquests. Mountains climbed, goals ticked off and new, bigger, better ones put in place; what a wonderful legacy for those around you.

I love to hear your stories, so please share them with me via email: info@lindasagementoring.com or on Facebook Linda Sage Mentoring; inspire others to dare, to achieve and to be, do, have everything that is their dream, just as you have now in your successful life.

Here's to your success in all the forthcoming years.

Caring for the Caregiver

ACKNOWLEDGEMENTS:

Muhammed Ali - January 17, 1942 – June 3, 2016

Quote "I'm not the greatest; I am the double greatest. Not only do I knock 'em out, I pick the round."

John McCarthy -27th November, 1956 (Longest held terrorist hostage, held in Lebanon for over 5 years)

Book: Some Other Rainbows

Quote: - 'I always thought it important to remember that the people holding me were human beings'

David Blunkett – 6th June, 1947

Book – On a Clear Day

Quote: - "I can hear people smile."

Andrea Bocelli - 22nd September, 1958

Quote: - "Like stars across the sky, we were born to shine"

Jim Rohn - September 17, 1930 – December 5, 2009
Quotes: - Skills – "Don't wish it were easier, wish you were better. Don't wish for less problems, wish for more skills. Don't wish for less challenges, wish for more wisdom.

Growth: - "Don't join an easy crowd, you won't grow. Go where the expectations and the demands to perform and achieve are high"

Change: - "We generally change ourselves for one of two reasons; inspiration or desperation"

Activity: - "The few who do, are the envy of the many who watch"

Success: - "Success is what you attract, by the person you become"

Henry Ford - July 30, 1863 – April 7, 1947

Quote: - "When everything seems to be going against you, remember that an aircraft takes off against the wind, not with it"

"Failure is simply the opportunity to begin again, this time more intelligently"

Douglas Bader - 21 February 1910 – 5 September 1982

Book – Reach for the Sky

Quote: - "Don't listen to anyone who tells you that you can't do this or that. That's nonsense. Make up your mind, you'll never use crutches or a stick, then have a go at everything. Go to school, join in all the games you can. Go anywhere you want to. But never, never let them persuade you that things are too difficult or impossible"

Sir Roger Gilbert Bannister, CH, CBE   23 March 1929 --

Book – The First Four Minute Mile

Quote: - "We run, not only because we think it is doing us good, but … because it helps us to do other things better"

ABOUT THE AUTHOR

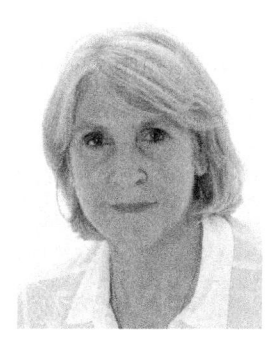

Linda Sage has worked for over thirty years in one field or another of self-development, working with the homeless to corporate executives. With her professional background in cognitive and behavioural psychology, Linda has covered many sectors within, health, wellbeing, education and entrepreneurship.

Her passion for personal growth and empowering personal achievement has covered many areas from personal change, to effective communications. No matter what you want to attain, or get better at in your life, personal change is essential. For your own business, for your career, for your relationships, for your financial security; staying the same and achieving something different is never going to work.

Linda has worked extensively in the UK, throughout Europe, the Middle East and America, her unwavering belief that all humans have buckets more potential than they will ever need or use inspires others to realize dreams/hopes/goals can come true and building your self-belief, self-accountability and self-discipline are the cornerstones to living the life you really want. There really are no limits on possibility, only the ones we impose on ourselves.

Linda mentors/coaches individuals, runs webinars, trains in companies and seminars, and writes numerous, books, blogs, articles and newsletters. As well as online training with video support, and numerous radio appearances, in many countries.

Linda has huge empathy and boundless energy to inspire, motivate and help people who want to make the most of their life. It is not to say that Linda's life has been effortless, she shares openly her personal stories of sadness and struggle; all of which have helped her in her own self-development. Linda says, "Life is a rollercoaster and sometimes we do not have control of the journey, but be most certainly do have control of how we react and respond to it. Hiding under the covers hoping it will pass us by, or by grabbing the reins and charging into adventure. Most people do not regret what they have done, or tried to do, but in later life, it is often the possibilities that were not taken, are most thought of."

To be, do and have whatever it is that you want in your life, is not selfish or self-centered, it is all about being the best person you can be in your life, and Linda believes that you can be working towards this every day, in each small choice, decision or action you do. Standing still in life is really not an option, but neither is it all about the end result; enjoy the journey, the people, the scenery and the memories along the way. The only conscience you have to live with, be at peace with is your own. Change is inevitable, each day, week, month or year for however long we have, so trying not to change is like trying to stop the tide come in, or the minutes passing.

Linda's future plans are to develop more online strategies and travel further afield with personal appearances, she is now based in England, and even with her hectic schedule, she is still involved in several charities for personal empowerment, anti-bullying and lifelong learning.

To get in touch with Linda, and find out more about what she does via her website

www.lindasage.com

or by email at info@lindasagementoring.com

You can also follow Linda on these platforms:

Facebook: https://www.facebook.com/lindasagementoring/

Linkedin: www.linkedin.com/in/linda-sage

YouTube: https://www.youtube.com/MeetLindaSage

Twitter: https://twitter.com/meetLindaSage

Linda can be booked for:

Personal Coaching

Corporate Training

Workshops

Seminars

Key Note Speeches

Caring for the Caregiver

Caring for the Caregiver

Printed in Great Britain
by Amazon